Nidotherapy

Harmonising the environment with the patient

Cheshire and Wirral Partnership NHS
NHS Foundation Trust

To Joan, Michael, Herman and Avis
who started it all off

Nidotherapy

Harmonising the environment with the patient

Peter Tyrer

RCPsych Publications

RCPsych Publications is an imprint of the Royal College of Psychiatrists,
17 Belgrave Square, London SW1X 8PG
http://www.rcpsych.ac.uk

British Library Cataloguing-in-Publication Data.
A catalogue record for this book is available from the British Library.
ISBN 978 1 904671 74 9

Distributed in North America by Publishers Storage and Shipping Company.

The views presented in this book do not necessarily reflect those of the Royal College of Psychiatrists, and the publishers are not responsible for any error of omission or fact.

The Royal College of Psychiatrists is a charity registered in England and Wales (228636) and in Scotland (SC038369).

Printed by Bell & Bain Limited, Glasgow, UK.

Contents

List of tables and boxes

Preface

This is a single author book, but nidotherapy is not the enterprise of a single person. Apart from the patients, whose contributions are seen clearly in many of the following pages, I owe a great deal to many who have allowed me to test out new approaches when an easier option would have been to say 'no', to others who have had the courage to go along with me as fellow nidotherapists and developed the approach in ways that were novel, perceptive and sensitive to patients' needs, to colleagues who may have looked askance at me at times for my personal eccentricities yet still offered gentle encouragement and support, and to the members of community teams who have to operate by consensus but still had shoulders broad enough to accommodate me without rejection. I must thank specifically Phil Harrison-Read, whose conversations over the years merged consensual management into nidotherapy, Peter Carter for defending my excesses, Helen Seivewright for showing that whatever determination and persistence I have is far exceeded by hers, Katarina Miloseška for reaching top speed faster than anyone I know from a standing start, Kofi Kramo for his cautious responses to my impulsive enthusiasm, Anna Maratos for showing that music therapy is the royal road to nidotherapy, Tom Sensky for showing that the measurement of treatment fidelity is far from a doddle, Maja Ranger for controlling her curiosity and ensuring all her research assessments were properly masked, Priya Bajaj for diligence beyond the call of any kind of duty, Catherine Gardiner, Ann-Marie Tully and Srjan Saso for the enthusiasm of youth and the promotion of drama, Derek Smith and Fergus O'Brien for putting us on film, Deirdre Dolan and Nancy Ababio for taking up the mantle assiduously without quite knowing what it was, Barbara Barrett for making me feel cost-effective, Sandra O'Sullivan for ensuring that every nidotherapy conference we mount lives up to its name, and Sarah-Jane Spencer for evaluating us with that mixture of engagement and independence that is the proper stuff of qualitative analysis.

I hope that all of these, together with the dozens of colleagues who have had to put up with my chuntering on the subject over the years, will recognise both the parts they have played in developing nidotherapy and at least some of its merits, and I reassure them that any faults and errors are entirely my own – but which I expect them to correct in due course.

Peter Tyrer

Foreword

It gives me enormous pleasure to write this foreword for Peter Tyrer's book on nidotherapy.

It is no surprise to me that Professor Tyrer is at the forefront of taking nidotherapy forward. Over many years Peter has pushed back the boundaries of psychiatry and has consistently brought lateral thinking to his clinical practice. Many of the concepts and techniques that he pioneered in the late '80s and early '90s are now embedded as mainstream practice in psychiatry not only in the UK but internationally.

I am therefore confident that nidotherapy will increasingly be adopted by clinicians throughout the spectrum of care ranging from nurses, occupational therapists, psychologists, social workers, psychiatrists and creative therapists such as art therapists and music therapists.

This book will be an essential aid to all of those interested in this therapy and I predict that not too many years from now nidotherapy will not only be in common use but will be seen as an essential tool in helping those with severe and enduring mental health problems in no lesser way that psychopharmacology is seen as an essential ingredient in current treatment.

I heartily commend this book.

Dr Peter Carter OBE
Chief Executive and General Secretary
Royal College of Nursing

Prologue

> I was also pleased that Dr Cawley, like myself, was interested in the Here and Now and not in theories about the past, and our talks were at first an accounting process, an examination of my emotional, personal, and even financial budget with a view to balancing all so that I could survive in spite of the bankruptcy imposed during my long stay in hospital, and my existence since then on unreal notions of myself, fed to me by myself and others, and now my sudden extreme poverty of being myself following the Investigation and the Verdict: the wastage of being other than myself could lead to the nothingness I had formerly experienced [Frame, 2001: p. 383].

Who is talking here, why should 'being myself' be thought of as a state of 'extreme poverty' and what on earth is the Investigation and the Verdict? These words come from the autobiography of Janet Frame (2001, first published in 1984). Janet was an aspiring writer who also acquired a less satisfactory label, a patient diagnosed with schizophrenia, in New Zealand in 1945. She came within a whisker of receiving a leucotomy in 1951, only receiving a reprieve at the last moment from Dr Blake Palmer, the physician superintendent at the hospital, when he noticed she had been awarded a national prize for her first book. 'I've decided you should stay as you are', he said, 'I don't want you changed'. She left hospital and went on a long search to find out whether the diagnosis she announced to her family, half with pride, half with fear, 'I've got Shizzophreenier', was true and what were its implications. This took her, not unsurprisingly at that time, to the psychiatric Mecca, the Maudsley Hospital in London, where she was assessed in great depth (the Investigation) and its conclusions given to her by Sir Aubrey Lewis (the Verdict). He concluded that she had never had schizophrenia and should never have been admitted to a mental hospital.

'The extreme poverty of being myself' came from the consequence of this revelation. 'The loss was great', she wrote, 'at first, the truth seemed to be more terrifying than the lie. Schizophrenia, as a psychosis, had been an accomplishment, removing ordinary responsibility from the sufferer. I was bereaved. I was ashamed. How could I ask for help directly when there was 'nothing wrong with me'?'(Frame, 2001: p. 375). Dr Robert Cawley, then a senior registrar later to become professor, provided this help in a series of treatment sessions with Janet, first as an in-patient and later as an out-patient when she obtained accommodation close to the hospital. Janet was, perhaps not surprisingly, generally antagonistic towards psychiatric methods and treatments, but Dr Cawley did not seem to have any special treatment to give. Janet was puzzled, and intrigued, and after a while there was progress.

> With time, the marvellous luxury of time, and patience, Dr Cawley convinced me that I was myself, I was an adult, I need not explain myself to others. The 'you should' days were over, he said. In his response to this lifelong urging of others to me that I should 'get out and mix', Dr Cawley was clear: his prescription for my ideal life was that I should live alone and write while resisting, if I wished this, the demands of others to 'join in' [p. 384].

Janet followed this path unerringly, became a highly acclaimed writer who was nominated for the Nobel Prize for Literature, and who has avoided the need for further psychiatric treatment after almost 10 years as an in-patient before she arrived at the Maudsley Hospital.

What was it that Dr Cawley, with Janet as a willing collaborator, achieved with this sensitive and sensitised young woman? My first post at the Maudsley Hospital in 1969 was as registrar to Dr Cawley and when I asked about his (already celebrated) treatment of Janet he described it as mainly 'listening to and understanding a very unusual person'. He told me he talked to her at length about complex equations, statistics and the evolution of species but very little about psychiatry. So why did she get better?

My guess, and I agree it can only be a guess, is that what helped her most was the administration of at least some of the aspects of nidotherapy (or nest therapy) (Tyrer, 2002). I agree this can only be speculation but both the account that Dr Cawley gave to me and the written words of Janet Frame give an outline to some of the essential features of nidotherapy described elsewhere in this book. These are very different from established psychotherapies and even though nidotherapy is included in a list of common psychotherapy procedures (http://www.commonlanguagepsychotherapy.org/) it is probably not a psychotherapy in the normal meaning of the term.

Some of the observations above are revealing. Janet was puzzled by the absence of therapy in Dr Crawley's intervention. 'Dr Cawley did not seem to have any special treatment to give, his sole triumph in our interviews was the accuracy of his recording the content'. Although the latter may have reflected the prevailing mood at the Maudsley Hospital at the time – 'record everything, however trivial it may appear to be, as amongst all the detritus you, or someone else, may detect pure gold' (Griffith Edwards, personal communication, 1969) – the absence of something identifiable as 'treatment' is a central feature of nidotherapy. This may appear to be a disadvantage but can be an asset with many patients who have been exposed to treatment for years and have concluded that, whatever its form, they do not like it. One of the initial advantages of the nidotherapist when approaching a patient is that they have no treatment to sell, no magic mix of jargon-loaded words that sound sensible at first but on reflection seem to have little substance, and which are all too often perceived by the patient, however unfairly, as a confidence trick to get them engaged.

Next, we have clues as to the content of the engagement. When Dr Cawley told me that his therapy was 'listening to and understanding a very unusual person' and that clearly this went on for many weeks, 'with time, the marvellous luxury of time, and patience', we can appreciate that what Dr Cawley did was to try and understand Janet as a person. This is often regarded as an essential component of many forms of psychotherapy, best summarised in the hackneyed phrase 'I can see where you're coming from' in response to disclosures from a patient. But this is not an understanding that can be derived from a single conversation. Nidotherapy attempts to discover all the places that people have come from, and a fair number of those they are going to, and not to use them in an exercise of know-all one-upmanship but to put them into a coherent pattern of aims, expectations and desires. Non-judgemental listening is another important part of nidotherapy, carried out not for the purpose of changing the person, but for getting to know them in the settings where they normally are or where they would like to be.

Next, Janet comments that Dr Cawley 'convinced me that I was myself, I was an adult, I need not explain myself to others'. This, I venture to suggest, is a common consequence of the systematic assessment of the environment that is a central part of nidotherapy. Most psychotherapies, however sensitive and careful they attempt to be, cannot help giving the impression to their clients that in some way they have been found wanting and need to be changed. Of course, most are willing accomplices in this transaction, as they too feel the need to change, but this acknowledgement is in itself a sign of failure. 'I was myself, I was an adult, I need not explain myself to others', are words pregnant with personal acceptance, the recognition that you are what you are, and not a person someone else would like you to be. What Janet saw as just 'accuracy in recording the content' of their interviews was probably a detailed assessment of the world as seen through Janet's eyes, not the therapist's own, nor her family (to whom she was very close), nor all those she had come to for advice over the years, but could truly reflect the words of Shakespeare's Othello, 'speak of me as I am, nothing extenuate' (*Othello*, Act V, Scene II). Such an analysis adopts the first principle of nidotherapy, something we have rather clumsily called 'collateral collocation' or 'setting the environmental requirements of patient and therapist(s) side by side and harmonising them' (Tyrer *et al*, 2003*a*). All of us, whether we are healthcare professionals, specialists in any field or just ordinary people, tend to be ready to give advice on what people should do, where they should live and how they should spend their time, particularly when these issues come into our area of special skills. We rarely go a stage further and find out exactly what is actually being perceived and interpreted by the individual when there is interaction, and sometimes collision, with the environment and its attendant consequences. Dr Cawley carried out this task with Janet in their long discussions, which incidentally would not be regarded as a cost-effective use of time in today's world of time-pressured, protocol-driven interventions, and so Janet's tribute to the 'marvellous luxury of time' is an apt one.

The consequence of the systematic assessment, exercised in full collaboration, was that Janet's view of the world, until then largely hidden except perhaps in her writings, was given proper prominence. It is fair to add that this is also an aim of some psychotherapies, but in nidotherapy it is obtained through the back door, as it were, by looking mainly at environmental influences. Robert Cawley would probably have included his intervention among the field of psychotherapies, albeit absent of a central defining structure, apart from what he described as the need for individual therapy. He later emphasised that the task of the psychiatrist is to 'recognise and make much of the uniqueness of the individual as well as the universality of scientific mechanisms', as psychiatry 'is alone in medicine in its primary concern with the multitudinous features which are unique for the individual' (Cawley, 1993: p. 155).

What followed the assessment was something like the process described in this book, beginning with an analysis of the environment from Janet's viewpoint, working out a set of targets and environmental changes (the nidopathway), and then letting her set forth in the confidence that she should celebrate herself and her talents without the corroding advice of others who knew her much less well than she did herself.

This book attempts to describe, organise systematically, help with training and plan what Janet Frame and Robert Cawley worked out together empirically, and many others attempt to do likewise, not always with the same degree of success. The selection of who should receive nidotherapy is a critical part of the process. Janet was diagnosed with schizophrenia at a time when a highly conventional society diagnosed many misfits as having the condition; a predilection carried to its ultimate excess by the new diagnosis of 'sluggish schizophrenia' in those unwise enough to express their dissidence in Soviet Russia. Now it is suggested Janet had high-functioning autism (Abrahamson, 2007), and though such a suggestion has been dismissed as nonsense by her family, one of whom has a child with autism, the simple fact that at present there is no adequate treatment for high-functioning autism and many other conditions within the autism spectrum disorders makes it ideal for nidotherapy. What Robert Cawley and Janet did together was to fashion a niche for a highly unusual person who was not fitting in to normal society, and in this niche she thrived and prospered.

We are not going to pretend that nidotherapy is complicated, requiring intellectual heavyweights for its practice and the need to be trained to perfection in a demanding programme. Some will say that its principles are those of holistic medicine they have practised all along, and others will claim it is common sense dressed up as science, but I would be very surprised if there was nothing that is perceived as new in the following pages. Where I accept our knowledge is very limited is in the milder degrees of mental illness, where lifestyle and symptoms overlap, and where nidotherapy probably has an important but as yet uncertain place (Tyrer, 2003). At the same time we make no apology for the focus made on those we have mainly treated with nidotherapy, the occupants of what one of our patients called 'the last chance saloon where only one of the exits leads on to health'.

These are early days. There are many improvements that can and must be made to the practice of and selection for nidotherapy and I end with an open invitation to contribute to this new development, an invitation that extends to all practitioners, carers and potential patients, as this is a genuine collaborative enterprise in which we can all become skilled. So please get in touch with us directly or through the nidotherapy website (www. nidotherapy.com) and help to keep us moving.

CHAPTER 1

General introduction and principles

Nidotherapy (the 'i' is long) is a treatment born of despair and desperation. It has been used to date mainly for a group of people with chronic mental illness who have been in the long-term care of psychiatric services in the UK. In describing this population it is necessary to put it into context. Before 1970 mental healthcare was generally split into two groups: a large group of patients in mental hospitals (asylums; it reached a maximum of 150 000 in 1964) who had major mental illness (psychoses, dementias and learning (intellectual) disability), many of whom stayed for many years, and another, larger group who were often characterised unfairly as the 'worried well' – as they were neither particularly worried nor particularly well – who lived in the community and were not generally stigmatised as being mentally ill, possibly because the full nature of their troubles was rarely admitted overtly. Most active psychiatric care was given to the second group, many of whom were classified as having either depression or neurotic or stress-related problems, and as much was given in public (National Health Service) as in private care. Of course treatment for the other group was also given, and there was some crossover between the two, but the treatment for the more severe psychoses was mainly pharmacological and given for those in psychiatric hospitals. Most of the new drug treatments had been introduced between 1950 and 1970 and for a time they were regarded with such high hopes that other treatments were lost in their shade (Sargant, 1966). Gradually, from about 1972 onwards, but only partly as a result of this new therapeutic optimism, the deinstitutionalisation of the mental hospital began, and those in the first hospital group (I will call it thus for short) were returned to the community in one form or another. Large institutions were regarded as bad and counter-therapeutic, and good community services, with a small institutional base linked to a clear geographical catchment area (Thornicroft & Tansella, 2004) were the new form of care for these patients. Oddly enough, the optimism behind this was so great that before long the term 'recovery' replaced 'rehabilitation' and 'long-term care' (see chapter 8) and the notion that no one with a mental illness should be regarded as immune from recovery became almost a politically correct mantra.

This pervasive optimism developed its own momentum. People were not allowed to rest under the label of any form of chronic mental illness. As Berrios has noted, a whole new vocabulary developed to fit this new attitude, which he summarised as psychiatric mercantilism:

> In the 'developed' Western world, 'treatment' and 'cure' are embedded in 'medical acts' which are being increasingly re-defined as scientific and mercantile transactions ('health' has become a 'commodity', patients 'clients', clinicians 'purveyors of health'). This new approach demands that the medical act be measured and priced and rendered economically efficient. Like the selling of faulty goods, 'lack of response' to treatment is increasingly being considered as a violation of a putative trade descriptions act. Courts need 'operational criteria' to decide on whether a breach of trust has occurred, and these are being provided by the so-called treatment guidelines which bodies of experts are increasingly compiling. Non-response to treatment can only be called 'treatment-resistance' if the guidelines have been complied with, and this lets the therapist off the hook. In social and legal terms, the notion of 'treatment resistance' can thus be used as an alibi as it transfers the responsibility for the lack of response from the therapist to the disease or the patient [Berrios, 2008: pp. 18–19].

So with this philosophy of care it is very difficult to admit to failure. In both the USA and the UK assertive community or outreach teams were introduced to cope with those who had not responded to conventional care, now rebranded as evidence-based psychiatry, to acknowledge that most standard interventions had been tested and had showed evidence of effectiveness, preferably in randomised trials.

This was the rocky terrain in which nidotherapy was developed. In the teams where it was practised there was no new therapy, only an enthusiastic model of care that involved teams from different disciplines and good collaborative working (Stein & Santos, 1998). But this was not always enough, and when the key purpose behind the introduction of these teams, a saving in the use of psychiatric beds, was not achieved (Burns *et al*, 1999; Harrison-Read *et al*, 2002; Killaspy *et al*, 2006) there was an urgent need to find something new. But when time after time each new therapy was thrown back as unacceptable or ineffective some radical changes in both approach and attitude were indicated.

This change was simple but dramatic. Instead of repeatedly trying to change people so that they fitted in better to their environments, we chose to change the environment so it made a better fit for the person. The adjustment of the environment is well exemplified by a bird's nest, a simple structure that adjusts to whatever is placed within it, and has the capacity to accommodate both large and small, multifaceted and round, sharp and blunt objects, and whether there are five fledglings or only one squawking within does not matter – it is equally suited to them all. We hypothesised that many people with the apparently intractable forms of mental illness seen in assertive outreach practice were out of harmony with their environment in all its forms, and it did not take too much to realise that many of them had pretty harsh and unforgiving surroundings that had never shown much degree of flexibility. This was the starting point of an approach which has developed considerably since the early days in 1988 when this therapy began, and which has moved far beyond its original context.

Theoretical basis of nidotherapy

We are all conscious of the importance of the environment in shaping our responses to the world. But although we stress the environment almost to excess during the phase of development when putting nature and nurture in head-to-head competitions with each other, we often forget about it when development has run its course and we have metamorphosed adults in a world where choice and control of the environment are taken for granted. So we seem as one with Shakespeare's Hamlet: 'What a piece of work is a man, how noble in reason, how infinite in faculties' (*Hamlet*, Act II, Scene II), a person who should have the capacity to fit the environment to his lofty aims without much in the way of assistance. But of course, we all tend to compete for the same things, and as Darwin demonstrated so convincingly in *The Origin of Species*, the struggle for dominance of the environment in competition with others is constant throughout life and across generations, and success comes to those who are best fitted for the environment. As he wrote: 'no country can be named in which all the native inhabitants are now so perfectly adapted to each other and to the physical conditions in which they live, that none of them could be still better adapted or improved' (p. 83) and consequently, 'the slightest advantage in certain individuals, at any age or during any season, over those with which they come into competition, *or better adaptation in however slight a degree to the surrounding physical conditions* (italics mine), will, in the long run, turn the balance' (Darwin 1859, reprinted 1970: p. 444). Nidotherapy is introduced, to rephrase Darwin's words again, to change the environment to create 'better adaptation in however slight a degree to the mental state conditions'. Thus with those who are persistently mentally ill, we should abandon the strategy of getting them to compete with others who are conventionally more fortunate and better able to compete, and instead attempt to match their special strengths with environments that suit them and which are not troubled by their weaknesses. So instead of having a large number of individuals competing for a limited space in the Sun we are creating a set of mini-environments, each fashioned to suit the person it is accommodating, not in competition with anyone else and which allows everyone to succeed. In a civilised world in which everyone is judged to have a place it is not appropriate to have everyone struggling for the same one, but in our pursuit of perfect health we recapitulate this stupidity. Darwin's principle of natural selection can be supplemented with the principle of nidotherapy, or 'informed environmental selection', 150 years after its publication in 1859.

Alpha children wear grey. They work much harder than we do, because they're so frightfully clever. I'm really awfully glad I'm a Beta, because I don't work so hard. And then we are much better than the Gammas and Deltas. Gammas are stupid. They all wear green, and Delta children wear khaki. Oh no, I don't want to play with Delta children. And Epsilons are still worse. They're too stupid ... [Huxley, 1932, reprinted in 2004: p. 75]

This is another way, described above shudderingly in Aldous Huxley's *Brave New World* in which children are deliberately bred to be different in their talents (Alpha at the top of the intellectual tree and Epsilon at the bottom) and then taught in their sleep (hypnopaedia) to prefer their group above all others. But this extreme of artificial selection has always remained a totalitarian fantasy and quite intolerable to those who wish for autonomy almost above all else and for whom Thomas Jefferson's unalienable rights of 'life, liberty and the pursuit of happiness' mean so much more than promises of spuriously more enticing rewards. Nidotherapy offers the same opportunity as that of people working side by side in life in reasonable harmony without the need for direct competition, a phenomenon known well in all civilised societies as the division of labour. But by concentrating on extending it to the environment in all its forms the division of labour becomes the division of living and not just confined to the workplace.

The parallels with Darwinian evolutionary theory should not be taken too far, as he was writing about competition over hundreds of generations, whereas the aim of nidotherapy is to create an immediate environmental shift. But although Darwin was enticed (by the psychologist Herbert Spencer) into adopting the phrase 'survival of the fittest' to summarise the main principle of evolution, he began by using the 'survival of the adapted', thereby stressing the important fit between organism and environment. This is the key to nidotherapy – it not only recognises that paying attention to the environment in mental health is valuable but goes further by arguing that the systematic planning and management of the environment is the best way to create mental harmony as a long-term goal.

Attitudes to treatment in mental illness

People who are ill are handicapped and want treatment to reverse the handicap. Do they really? How often have you asked them? It is true of many, but not all, physical disorders, but certainly not the norm in many forms of mental illness. The uninformed visitor observing clinical practice in mental health services is often very surprised by the lack of interest in treatment. Those with the most severe mental illnesses, the psychoses, a spectrum that crosses from bipolar disorder to schizophrenia, are often remarkable in their antipathy to anything being delivered to them in the guise of therapy. I well remember a young man with schizophrenia who developed an inoperable tumour and slowly wasted away as the cancer took hold. But he almost ignored his bodily decay; everything seemed to be subsumed to his burning desire to be rid of antipsychotic drug treatment for his schizophrenia. His wish in his final days was to go home to his family and no longer be detained under the Mental Health Act, and both were granted. Three weeks later he became very agitated by difficulty in breathing and I brought some diazepam to him at home to try and relieve these symptoms. As I gave the little box of tablets to him he sat up suddenly, gripped my arm and staring at me, said triumphantly, 'I don't have to take these, you know, because I'm not under a section now.' He died 2 days later having taken only one of these tablets; he remained consistent to the last.

This is not an isolated account of antipathy. Although they are clearly a selected group, most people who are in-patients in psychiatric wards are either ambivalent or hostile to treatment, no matter its nature. One of the standard explanations for this is that the most effective treatments for the manic phase of bipolar disorder and the positive symptoms of schizophrenia are the antipsychotic drugs, and these often attract the title 'dirty drugs' because of their wide range of adverse effects (it is no coincidence that the first of these, chlorpromazine, was called Largactil because of the large number of pharmacological actions it possessed). Unfortunately we remain with dirty drugs for psychoses as the newer versions just have a different range of adverse effects that give them no special advantages (Leucht et al, 2009).

It might be thought that antipathy to the adverse effect of these drugs was the reason for poor adherence to treatment, but other interventions for these conditions are equally unpopular. Cognitive–behavioural therapy was introduced for the treatment of schizophrenia 15 years ago and has been demonstrated to be of value, at least in the short term (Kingdon & Turkington, 1995; Tarrier et al, 1999), but its effects are not long-lasting and it has limited value in preventing relapse (Garety et al, 2008). What is more disturbing is that only a minority of people volunteer for the treatment and adhere to it. As Jan Scott (2008) has summarised the evidence with regard to schizophrenia, 'the world of routine psychiatric practice brings us into contact with some patients who do not want or do not respond optimally to antipsychotic medication, but who also do not always want or benefit from psychological therapies either.' When given the opportunity, is it not curious that only a minority of patients volunteer for a treatment that might lead to at least a reduction in the dosage of the antipsychotic drugs they are so keen to avoid?

This lack of enthusiasm for treatment is commonly put down to an absence of insight or sometimes an absence of capacity. If someone is not aware they are ill it is not surprising that they see no need for any remedy. But there are other reasons that cannot be put at the door of the illness and its direct effects. One of the reasons why patients are so dissatisfied with current therapeutic delivery systems is that they are perceived as making them into people they are not. Of course, if their symptoms improve with treatment and they recognise the advantages of these changes there is no problem with persisting with treatment as adherence is likely to be good. But many others do not improve quite in the same way; they want to be different in their general functioning but not in the way the services expect.

In addition, some people with long-standing disability such as personality disorder, intellectual disability and chronic psychosis, have accepted the way they are and feel that if they were more comfortable in their surroundings in all its physical and personal forms they would not need to have treatment for what other people, looking at the problem from a perspective quite different from that of the patient, regard as an intractable mental disorder.

The argument that various happenings and circumstances are the cause of problems with mental health is nothing new. A whole field of research has developed out of life events research and yet another into post-traumatic stress disorder that is now so well-developed some think of it as an industry. However, interventions for these disorders are focused on helping people to adjust to events and turbulency, not on changing the environment in a substantial and permanent way. Even those treatments that have been focused primarily on the environment – whether it be bed rest following myocardial infarction, sanatoria in the high Alps for those with tuberculosis, or light therapy for seasonal affective disorder – are making temporary and short-term changes to the environment only. Nidotherapy attempts to make a more permanent change. Sometimes this can overlap with direct treatment; one of our patients with seasonal affective disorder found out that he remained well if he visited members of his family in New Zealand in the UK winter, and decided eventually to go to New Zealand every year to keep his mood in good order (Tyrer *et al*, 2003a).

Although we live in an age that proclaims the advantages of diversity, we are in danger of becoming slaves to approved fashions and are increasingly intolerant of variety we do not share, which is especially true with much of the diversity demanded by the mentally ill. Nidotherapy acknowledges diversity in a more honest and open way than most other approaches. Dr Cawley persuaded Janet Frame to admit something she knew all along, 'I was myself, I was an adult, I need not explain myself to others', but over the years of conventional psychiatric treatment she had been told repeatedly that she was abnormal, even to the extent of having prefrontal leucotomy recommended, so it is not surprising she had begun to doubt her own beliefs. Many other patients, either suffering alone or in long-term psychiatric care, are in the same position as Janet. They feel they know themselves but are repeatedly told that this knowledge is defective, that they should be looking for a different person that 'therapy', whatever is nature, will enable them to discover.

Fundamental differences between nidotherapy and other psychotherapies

Although the differences between nidotherapy and other psychotherapies are addressed in more detail later in this book, it is also worth stressing them at this point. Nidotherapy is not just a form of environmental manipulation or social engineering, a social model of psychiatry (Tyrer & Steinberg,

2005) that regards most interventions in mental illness as examples of 'medicalising'. Such a model does indeed focus on the social environment but generally makes no attempt to change it specifically as a form of management. Nidotherapy is also none of the following: a rebadged housing advice service or accommodation bureau; a career development service that finds out your abilities and picks the right role; a lifestyle advisory service or an internet dating service that provides the perfect place to meet the person of your dreams (although it is prepared to use any of these agencies once a way forward (nidopathway) has been developed). Instead, it is essentially a complicated matching process whereby people's deep desires, vague wishes, fundamental opinions and lifestyle are understood sufficiently to ensure that environmental factors in all their forms are adjusted sensitively and specifically to make the best fit for the patient. There are many other treatments that take great account of the environment but they are all fundamentally concerned with making adjustments to the person, either exclusively or sometimes in connection with the environment, but in which all environmental changes are made to facilitate the person changes. Such treatments include person-centred planning, cognitive–behavioural therapy, modelling and shaping, schema-focused therapy, family therapy, systems theory, social case work and the care programme approach.

So in strict terms, nidotherapy is not a treatment because its prime purpose is to manipulate the environment or promote a better engagement with it, and any changes in the patient are secondary to this manipulation. When nidotherapy crosses the border into direct treatment of the patient it is no longer nidotherapy and can use any of the psychotherapeutic interventions described above. Quite often there is an element of nidotherapy in conventional mental health services, particularly when a clinical team gets to the point of saying 'Nothing has worked so far, what do we do now?' At this point of fitting a square peg into a round hole, therapists can sometimes take more interest in the hole than the peg. Even when it does get to this point there is a tendency to adopt a paternalistic approach in which the patient is a passive onlooker and the general attitude is 'You stay out of this for the time being. We'll sort out what you need and then let you know.' Often good environmental changes are being made at these times, but it is much better to have them recognised clearly instead of relying on 'sleep-walking nidotherapy' in which some aspects of the treatment are being used but neither patient nor therapist know what they are doing and why.

So the important questions to ask yourself if you are doing something that may or may not be nidotherapy are best expressed as:

1   Is the considered intervention designed to change the patient's environment in the long term?
2   Is the change designed specifically to promote the patient's environmental adjustment?

It is only when both are answered positively that we can conclude that nidotherapy is being practised. The other therapies described above are all designed to change *people*, and although the environment may often be altered in these therapies, it is done as part of the treatment of the person.

The division between nidotherapy and other treatments is therefore straightforward. When nidotherapy crosses the border into direct treatment of the patient it is no longer nidotherapy, and when other forms of treatment cross from being patient-centred to entirely environment-centred they may become nidotherapy. It is useful to give an example from our practice to illustrate this. A patient whose main problem was obsessional hoarding used to carry a great many polythene bags with him when he went to the local supermarket. He was regarded as a hazard with all these bags and was banned from shopping there. When assessed by his nidotherapist he identified the difficulty of going to the supermarket as one of the environments he would like to visit. After negotiation he was persuaded to put his goods into only two bags and with these he was granted access to the supermarket again. Some would say this was an example of behaviour therapy with possible cognitive overtones but the behaviour had not changed in any fundamental way; it was just that many bags of apparent rubbish were converted into two bags and this was deemed acceptable. More importantly, the patient regarded it as a victory as all his hoarding principles had not been compromised in any way. The difference is subtle but relevant – if he had been persuaded that it was wise to take fewer possessions into the supermarket as he would have an obvious gain, this would have been behaviour therapy. The small difference is important; the environment had changed a little, the patient had not.

Ego-dystonicity and ego-synchronicity

Ego-dystonicity and ego-synchronicity were described by the psychoanalyst Franz Alexander more than three-quarters of a century ago (Alexander, 1930). Symptoms and behaviours that are ego-syntonic are consistent with the person's normal functioning and regarded as integral. Those that are ego-dystonic are viewed as alien and undesirable and so are desired to be removed as soon as possible. Sometimes the same symptom can be present in both groups. For most people the symptom of depression is ego-dystonic but when it becomes part of an integrated view of the world it may be ego-syntonic. Most nidotherapy is best suited to problems that are ego-syntonic – the ones that are problems to others but not to those who experience them, who tend to regard the difficulties created as caused by those who complain rather than by they themselves.

Of course there is bound to be overlap between nidotherapy and other forms of psychological treatment and it does no particular good to spend time quibbling over whether an intervention is really one therapy or another. The essential differences between nidotherapy and other forms of management are summarised in Table 1.1, but the underlying philosophy is at the core of all these differences. The nidotherapist takes people as they are and not as individuals who desire to be changed, and the challenge of 'treatment'

Table 1.1 Essential differences between nidotherapy and other psychological therapies

Essentials of nidotherapy	Essentials of other psychotherapies
Environment-centred	Person-centred
Makes no attempt to change the person	Directly or indirectly attempts to improve the person through change
Attempts to promote adaptation by selecting suitable environments	When attempting to promote adaptation does so in the context of helping the person to adjust better
Close relationship with person needed to understand environmental needs	Relationship with person developed to aid understanding and treatment of psychological problems
Aims to make the person feel more at home in every sense	Aims either to relieve the person of unpleasant symptoms or distress or to understand the person more
Collaboration at the environmental level allows the person to choose the most fitting of living settings	Collaboration, when promoted, is used as a means to effect personal change

is to reach the harmony of 'perfect person–setting concordance', or the ideal environment to match the needs of the person. This is the philosophy of adaptation, not of change, and it differs from all other psychological therapies in this regard. So when asking yourself whether something you do is nidotherapy or something else, just ask 'Am I doing this because I want to change this attitude, symptom, behaviour or need, or am I accepting this as part of the person and want to accommodate it?' It is clear which is the path to nidotherapy.

CHAPTER 2

Assessing the patient for nidotherapy

We hope the previous chapter has made it clear that nidotherapy is not just another form of conventional psychotherapy that follows a set of principles aimed at changing the person in treatment. It requires a new understanding of the setting where the problem lies that is not merely used as a vehicle to understand the problem better (which it most certainly should if it goes well) but then becomes the prime mover in changing the environment in all its forms. The following example illustrates one of the key aspects of the treatment – environmental understanding, and although it is a simple one, it must be familiar to hundreds of health professionals who come across angry people who have just been admitted to hospital compulsorily. Nidotherapy requires us to know the setting and so we have first to set the scene. The example (Case study 2.1*a*) is a very common one for those who are currently practising in hospital settings.

Case study 2.1a

Scene: Day room of a psychiatric ward in a general hospital. The room is new but already the plastic chairs are ingrained with coffee and food stains and both the staff and patients carry out their activities with a general desultory air indicating something less than full enthusiasm. A junior psychiatrist (Dave) has just been allocated to a new post and is going round to meet all the patients on his list. He is interviewing Fred, who has a diagnosis of schizophrenia and is unwillingly in hospital on a compulsory order.

Dave: 'How long have you been in hospital now?

Fred: 'You don't need to ask me that – just look in those notes', indicating the clinical notes brought in by Dave and left on the table.

Dave (trying another tack): 'How are you feeling now?'

Fred: 'Fed up because you're bothering me.'

Dave: 'There's no point in acting like that. I'm trying to help you but you won't help me.'

> **Case study 2.1a** *(contd)*
>
> Fred: 'You're not trying to help me. You're just like all the rest. You just want to get me to talk to you so I say something stupid and give you an excuse to give me another injection and stop me leaving the hospital. I'm not *** well going to give you the pleasure; I'm clearing off now.'
>
> Fred walks out of the room and slams the door. Dave shakes his head, goes out to the nursing station where the notes are kept and discusses the difficult interview he has had with the nursing staff. They confirm that he has been antagonistic towards them all day and spends most of the day on his own looking furtively at others but having very little contact with them, including the refusal to take part in all group activities. Dave's opinion is reinforced and he writes in Fred's file:
>
> 'Remains hostile and paranoid. Will not engage in sensible discussions. May need to increase medication if he does not improve.'
>
> What is missing here?

I am not criticising Dave for doing what he has done, because in the language of today, his assessment of Fred is perfectly proper. His suggestion of an increase in medication could be described as 'evidence-based' as the most effective treatment for schizophrenia is an antipsychotic drug in the lowest possible dose that suppresses symptoms, although even that is looking a little shaky as the handicaps of antipsychotic drugs become more prominent. I also feel it right to emphasise that even if Dave had gone out of his way to be especially pleasant to Fred it would have been still just as likely that he would have reacted in the same way. This is because Fred is likely to be genuinely paranoid, not just upset because he is in hospital against his will, as paranoid delusions, or baseless beliefs held with very strong conviction, are among the key features of schizophrenia, and he is liable to misinterpret any form of positive engagement as a ruse to put him off his guard. In deciding what is missing in Dave's evaluation of Fred let us try and guess how each of them interprets the different elements of their recent encounter (Table 2.1).

Table 2.1   Consequences of environmental misunderstanding

Perceived problem	Dave's and hospital staff's interpretation	Fred's view
Refusal to talk to staff in hospital	This is consistent with his paranoia – he doesn't trust anybody and he's probably hearing voices	There's no point in talking to them. They've locked me up in here and are going to do exactly as they please
Hostility whenever approached by staff	This man is aggressive. We must check our risk management strategy to protect ourselves and others	I'm frightened of these people and angry with them at the same time. I don't know how to handle them and wish they would go away

Table continues

11

Table 2.1   *Continued*

Perceived problem	Dave's and hospital staff's interpretation	Fred' sview
Withdrawal and non-cooperation with ward activities	This man's schizophrenia makes him unable to relate to others, so he spends all his time alone	I don't know the people here, I don't belong, so why should I talk to anyone?
Appears to be abnormally suspicious	It is likely that he has paranoid delusions and this explains his suspicions as he believes he is being persecuted	I've been forced here against my will and have no idea what's going to happen next – injections, tablets, a locked ward – anybody would be suspicious in my situation

What is missing in Dave's evaluation is an appreciation of what Fred feels in this situation and how it might be explored in a constructive way. We do not know from the accounts in Table 2.1 whose interpretation is correct. Fred may be a very suspicious person with a host of strange experiences and beliefs that merit an increase in medication, but he could also be as normal as anybody can claim to be in this day and age, and all his so-called pathological behaviour could be explained entirely by his situation. Dave does not know which of these explanations is correct because he has made no attempt to achieve environmental understanding. What he could, indeed should, have done is to talk to Fred in a different way to at least allow an alternative explanation to be put on the diagnostic table. Let us assume that Fred does not have any form of psychosis now and his views are actually the right ones. This is how Dave could have elicited this (Case study 2.1*b*).

It does not need much imagination to realise from this conversation that whatever was the problem last night it is not present now and before long Fred and Jackson are likely to be reunited.

Now let us take another scenario. Let us assume that Fred has indeed got paranoid schizophrenia, has been on all the treatments known for the condition and has not shown any significant response. What do we do if there is no other treatment in the offing for him and he is deemed just to have chronic schizophrenia? The first part of nidotherapy just described can now be extended to a full nidotherapy assessment as his condition is stable but the outcome is unsatisfactory and nothing more of assistance seems to be planned.

These examples show the difficulty that many practitioners (and indeed patients) have in deciding when is the right time to stop treating the patient or, as a nidotherapist puts it, ceasing to change the person and starting to change the environment. We live in an age in which every ill is considered treatable and so when someone does not respond the term 'treatment-resistant' is used, even though the possibility that the treatment is not appropriate could be an equally good explanation. The advocates of the treatment-resistant concept will go on repeatedly attempting to introduce

Case study 2.1b

We will start the conversation as before.

Dave: 'How long have you been in hospital now?

Fred: 'You don't need to ask me that – just look in those notes', indicating the clinical notes brought in by Dave and left on the table.

Dave (trying another tack): 'How are you feeling now?'

Fred: 'Fed up because you're bothering me.'

Dave: 'I can quite see that. I think I'd feel fed up too if I was in your position. It's no joke being admitted to hospital against your will.'

Fred: 'OK then, so why not discharge me?'

Dave: 'I can't discharge you on my own; I'm only the junior doctor in the team. But I can help, if I can find out from you how you really are at present. I can quite understand why this place makes you feel angry and annoyed; it would make me frightened as well, but I want to know if you would feel exactly the same if you were somewhere else, say back at home?'

Fred: 'There you are, then. Try it out. Let me go home and I'll see you there.'

Dave: 'So you would be quite happy seeing me at home then. What's it like there?'

Fred: 'Nothing much to write home about. But it's OK for me. I've got a computer that I use all the time and I've a cat too who keeps me good company.'

Dave: 'A cat! I like cats too. What's his name?'

Fred: 'Jackson. I named him after that character in Beatrix Potter who never wipes his feet. He's only got one eye but he makes sure it rests on me when he wants something.'

Dave: 'Who's looking after him now then?'

Fred: 'That's one of the reasons I want to get back home. I don't know what happened last night – I honestly don't recall a thing – but I need to get back home and feed him because he'll be starving'.

old, new and untried treatment for the condition on the basis that it is a disorder and therefore must be treated. In making this decision we need to be reminded that almost all psychiatric disorders are fictional representations of common presentations of mental illness; they are not disorders in any other sense and the biological underpinnings of many of the diagnoses are still imperfect.

Once the therapist moves over from 'treatment-resistant' to 'state acceptance' matters change greatly. It is not that all attempts are made to abandon treatment – indeed, any existing treatment can be continued – but a deliberate decision is made to accept the person for what they are and assume, perhaps pessimistically but often realistically that nothing essential is going to change for the foreseeable future. This can often be perceived as a release by the patient; the quest for the holy grail of cure has stopped and a reappraisal of everything else can now begin.

Who should carry out the assessment for nidotherapy?

Assessments for nidotherapy can be carried out by a range of professionals and non-professionals (including patients themselves) but with the more severe mental disorders it is unwise to proceed without expert professional help. This does not mean that once a patient has been selected by a professional for nidotherapy they cannot be treated by someone with relatively little knowledge of severe mental illness (see chapter 7), but the important decision of when nidotherapy should be introduced can only be made by people with significant knowledge of the nature and course of the mental illnesses concerned. If there is no concurrent mental illness requiring, or even being considered for, treatment, then there is no special need for high-quality professional input and in self-nidotherapy (see chapter 6) the decisions can be made entirely by the person concerned.

Which disorders might be treated with nidotherapy?

Minor disorders

The term 'minor mental illness' is a misnomer, but it covers most of the common conditions called adjustment disorders (abnormal reactions to life events), anxiety and depression, and many phobic, obsessional and eating disorders. These are often not minor and cause a great deal of suffering over a long period, but the adjective is used to distinguish them from major mental illness (see below).

Most people with these so-called minor disorders are fully aware of their problems and the difficulties they are causing; indeed they are often experts in their own condition when it has been persisting or recurring for many years. These conditions also include what are frequently called the cluster C personality disorders (the anxious–fearful cluster) in which the person has persistent worries, mixtures of anxiety and depression, fears of impending catastrophe and a range of behaviours, including obsessional ones, to attempt to preserve a state of equilibrium.

Many people with these disorders decide themselves to change their lifestyle in an attempt to achieve greater life satisfaction. What can be called the 'Scottish croft' syndrome, the desire to escape a high-pressured but lucrative existence in an adverse environment in place of an idyllic one (a Scottish croft) with a much less pressured and satisfying lifestyle is an example of this syndrome. Sometimes it works, sometimes it does not, but in most cases the people concerned do not seek special advice before making these decisions. They discuss it among friends and colleagues and decide, often after agonising about financial issues for many months, whether or not such a move is desirable and feasible. The reason why it is worth calling this a syndrome is that it frequently does not succeed because the very characteristics that have led to success in the adverse environment are taken to the new one and may be reused with the same consequences. Of course the opposite can happen and the new life does indeed become an idyllic one, often cushioned by the financial rewards from the previous existence.

In such cases the individuals wanting nidotherapy can make these decisions almost on their own, although often their general practitioner may be involved in helping to come to such a decision.

Major mental illnesses

The conditions subsumed under the category of major mental illness include the schizophrenia–bipolar spectrum covering the range of psychotic disorders, from frank and unequivocal schizophrenia through to schizoaffective psychoses and bipolar disorder (Craddock & Owen, 2005), in which both manic and depressed phases of the condition are present at different times. It also includes the organic disorders of dementia and acquired brain injury through trauma or other reasons (e.g. alcohol misuse). In these disorders the illness has major effect on all aspects of functioning and is illustrated by a name sometimes given to the most serious forms of these disorders, disintegrative psychoses.

These conditions are generally treatable but approximately 5 to 10% of individuals thus diagnosed do not respond to any significant degree and another large proportion have other pathologies that make their recovery only partial. The recurring difficulty in assessing such people is that despite often having clear wishes and aims, they lack the capacity possessed by those with minor mental illnesses to make sound and reasoned judgements that can influence the choice of therapy. This is far from saying that the individual concerned should be ignored in this decision-making; it is just that the broad perspective necessary to make what are in effect major changes in peoples' lives and management can often not be assessed dispassionately and choices made easily by the individuals concerned. The development of coercive measures in every country in the world in the form of mental health legislation illustrates this problem. When people are not able to make cogent assessments of their mental state, others, at least in the short term, have to do it for them.

The nidotherapist in these instances is put in a difficult position. If they rely on the patient's expressed views alone, things can go badly wrong. Thus, for example, a very large number of people with the most common psychotic disorder, paranoid schizophrenia, would like to be left alone to work out solutions for themselves without the need for regular antipsychotic medication. This wish is understandable at one level as the main treatments for schizophrenia are pharmacological, with a range of side-effects that are far from pleasant, but at another level the recognition of illness and its presence is often defective (commonly expressed as lack of insight) and what the patient perceives as an excellent way forward is seen by others, on the basis of the person's observed behaviour, as catastrophically inappropriate.

A great number of patients with schizophrenia could therefore present with a request for nidotherapy. 'Hugs, not drugs', a common chant in the anti-psychiatry movement, can be extended to 'Give me an environmental hug and my schizophrenia will go away'. Of course, this is not the case, but there is a point in the treatment of major psychoses where continuing treatment feels like hitting your head against a brick wall, there is much pain but no gain and something else has to be tried. This is the territory where nidotherapy may be helpful. It is not given as an alternative to other treatments in these circumstances, but if successful, it may reduce the need for at least some of these therapies because it promotes better adaptation and adjustment.

The well-known and influential research of George Brown, Julian Leff and others (Brown & Harris, 1978; Leff *et al*, 1982) has demonstrated the adverse effects of life events in triggering a wide range of psychiatric disorders, including evidence that high-expressed emotion can generate and promote relapse in schizophrenia. This illustrates the importance of the environment, and change in this in the form of reduction of expressed emotion is associated with a lower need for antipsychotic drugs (Leff *et al*, 1985). (However, and we shall see that later, nidotherapy attempts to go much further than just removing a single negative aspect of the environment as it promotes new adaptive ones).

The decision when to stop treating a major mental illness on the grounds that it is no longer treatment-resistant but 'treatment-unproductive' is not an easy one. Ideally it should be decided by the therapist involved in treating the major psychosis before making a referral for nidotherapy, but in some instances it would have to be decided by the nidotherapy team after a full initial assessment.

Personality disorder

Nidotherapy was first introduced for people who had 'personality disorders' (Tyrer, 2002). This term is put in quotes because it is an unsatisfactory and pejorative label. It describes a group of conditions that are not classical disorders but are better described as diatheses, or persistent tendencies which in varying degrees make the person more vulnerable to problems in life including the development of various mental illnesses (Tyrer, 2007). They very frequently co-occur with other mental illness and complicate treatment in progress (Newton-Howes *et al*, 2006). This is because the personality, or characteristic style of behaving, of the individuals concerned complicates management. These conditions are remarkably common in mental health services and the general rule is that the further you go in a psychiatric referral system the more likely you are to have a personality problem (Tyrer, 2008). Only about 35% of patients referred to mental health services have such problems, but in tertiary referral services such as assertive outreach teams the prevalence of personality problems rises to over 90% (Ranger *et al*, 2004).

Personality diathesis covers a range of abnormalities from personality difficulties through to severe personality problems or disorder. The distinction between what is disorder and what is difficulty is entirely an arbitrary one and this explains the advantages of the word diathesis, which could describe abnormality as a set of different levels of severity without ever referring to the word 'disorder'.

There are several reasons why those with personality problems are well suited to nidotherapy:

1   there are relatively few effective treatments for personality problems in evidence-based psychiatry, with only borderline personality disorder showing any real suggestion of efficacy (Bateman & Zanarini, 2008),

2   most of those with personality problems do not wish to receive treatment for them (Tyrer *et al*, 2003*b*), and

3   the problems tend to be persistent.

This last characteristic needs to be qualified. Personality problems, whether described as difficulty, disorder or psychopathy, fundamentally involve impaired relationships with other people. When the environment is adverse to the problems of the particular personality, then the personality function is disordered, though this could quickly change when the environment becomes more conducive to that personality style. Thus, for example, a person with an obsessive eye for detail may perform extremely badly in an entrepreneurial environment where controlled risk-taking is necessary, but perform much more effectively in a well-established structure where there are clear rules and planned patterns of behaviour that have been shown to produce success. In such instances the person may appear to be disordered in personality function at one moment and very shortly afterwards appears to be adaptive. However, the underlying personality has not changed fundamentally and it is this that is likely to be persistent rather than what can be described as 'personality function' (Tyrer *et al*, 2007), the day-to-day expression of overt behaviour including any difficulties in relationships with others.

It is therefore those who have personality diatheses and other persistent disorders that may represent the best opportunity for nidotherapy, but as this subject is a special personal interest I could be wrong. Nidotherapy was originally introduced for such patients in our clinical services. Those who have been treated were those in whom all active therapeutic endeavour had more or less ceased and the teams concerned were carrying out a holding operation in trying to prevent further damage rather than promoting any therapeutic change. It is when therapists have reached this point with any long-standing problem that the nidotherapy approach is worth considering.

Personality as the centre of nidotherapy

In emphasising the role of changing the environment in nidotherapy it is wrong to assume that this is a straightforward exercise in which the patient feeds information to the therapist that is then used to make the environmental change. At the heart of nidotherapy is the Darwinian concept of adaptation. However, it is not the blind adaptation of random changes in successive generations of the person controlled by the selfish gene in its quest for domination (Dawkins, 2006), but a controlled and subtle adaptation of the surroundings so that the misfit is reclaimed and becomes a good fit. This cannot be done by ticking a set of boxes in an interview format because very few people are able to decide on what their perfect environmental match would be. The Sanskrit term nirvana is probably the best example of the ultimate in nidotherapy, 'an ideal condition of rest, harmony, stability, or joy', or absolute harmony with the physical, social and personal environment. I know nobody who has claimed to have reached this state despite excessive trying.

Approaching close to this idealised goal cannot be achieved without a really good understanding of the person whose environmental needs are being assessed. This needs an understanding of personality function; good, adequate and poor function, in all areas of existence. Personality represents the interaction between the person and the environment, and personality disorder is the most prominent form of mismatch, so it is not an accident that this group of conditions figures strongly in nidotherapy. But I stress again that 'personality disorder' is wrongly named; it implies a long-lasting or even permanent abnormality of function. This is why it has become such a pejorative word in mental health, where it is wrongly assumed to carry the additional label of 'untreatable'. But many with personality disorder lose their disorders without any apparent treatment. It can be argued that their personalities have changed spontaneously, but in many cases their personalities have not altered; instead, the environment has.

Patricia Cohen and her colleagues at the University of Columbia, New York, gathered evidence of this in a detailed follow-up of a community sample of 629 adolescents first interviewed at 14 years of age and then up to 19 years later in the Children in the Community Study. The study has shown that people with evidence of both personality and mental state disturbance in adolescence fare worse than those without these problems (or one only) (Crawford et al, 2008a) but many still improve and lose all their symptoms. What has been noted by Cohen and her colleagues (Cohen, 2006) is that some of those with persistent personality difficulties show a substantial decline in these long-term serious problems for no apparent reason. However, when they looked at these people in more detail it was clear that what had happened was that the environments had changed, not the people. Thus, for example, a person with chronic employment difficulties who had been sacked many times from jobs because of insubordinate behaviour and whose life was in constant chaos, suddenly settled with a steady job and good relationships with all. He had simply found a job that suited his personality, had improved his self-esteem enormously, and the pieces of the jigsaw in the rest of his life had all slotted into place. Even though the Children in the Community Study was not concerned with any particular intervention, Dr Cohen had suggested the name 'niche therapy' for what had happened to this person (Cohen, 2006), after the work by Willi (1999).

Of course, nidotherapy is niche therapy; both Latin and French words refer to the nest.

The task of nidotherapy is to fashion and plan the niche rather than just let it occur by chance, as when these sudden improvements occur they are very seldom planned. They cannot usually be planned because the person at the centre of the action does not know what change is needed, and all too often people are telling them that it is them who need to change.

Choosing the time to start nidotherapy

As already indicated, it is unwise to start nidotherapy when a new or enhanced treatment is being tested. Just as it is not wise to introduce psychological treatments for anxiety in the middle of a series of investigations for a serious physical illness, it is similarly best to wait until a new treatment has had an adequate chance to show its benefits before a different approach is tried. The outcome of some disorders can change greatly with a revolutionary new treatment – one of the best examples is the treatment of resistant schizophrenia with clozapine – but there is no point in effecting a permanent environmental change if the person is going to alter to such an extent that that change either becomes unnecessary or completely inappropriate.

If the mental disorder manifest by the patient is temporary, or has an excellent chance of being resolved without a specific treatment, there is also little point in introducing nidotherapy unless there is additional pathology. A series of adjustments made to counteract the handicap of a mental difficulty may look impressive at first, but if the mental difficulty goes away, so does the reason for the intervention.

There is also the need to get the agreement of the patient for intervention. We have already indicated that many people with persistent illness are only too pleased to have the opportunity to take part in an enterprise that accepts them as they are, but there are many others who are very sceptical. A response equivalent to 'A plague on all your houses – you've given me this treatment and that treatment and made promise after promise, but I'm still no better off. Why should I listen to a single word you say?' is far from uncommon. 'Treatment-resistant' often means 'therapist-resistant' also, and in chapter 4 ways of getting round this problem in nidotherapy are described. But in the last resort the patient has to come to the nidotherapy table at some point in treatment; so it is right to get at least some of the elements of cooperation early in the process of assessment.

Intervention in nidotherapy may also be delayed by procrastination of the patient even when it seems quite clear to all involved that environmental change is needed. One of the many reasons why so many people fail to take advantage of nidotherapy is that they are suffering from what might be called the 'Prufrock syndrome', named after the well-known poem by T. S. Eliot (1917). This is a state of general dissatisfaction with life caused by self-perpetuated environmental restriction, and is just ripe for nidotherapy. J. Alfred Prufrock can only be identified through the words of the poem but is clearly a man at the wrong end of middle age – 'I grow old… I grow old…, I shall wear the bottoms of my trousers rolled' – who is lonely and dissatisfied with his lot in life but apparently powerless to do anything about it. His 'Love Song', not a song at all, is an ironic description of his wish to break outside an obsessional, miserable, unnoticed existence – but which is thwarted by his lack of confidence and poor self-esteem. He wants to develop relationships that would enrich his life, preferably with a feisty female, but his weak attempts to do so are throttled by doubt almost before they begin.

> And indeed there will be time
> To wonder, 'Do I dare?' and, 'Do I dare?'

He meets a group to have 'toast and tea' and in this genteel setting he ponders on how to contribute, but of course ends up in reflective paralysis:

> Do I dare
> Disturb the universe?
> In a minute there is time
> For decisions and revisions which a minute will reverse.

But this is not just an isolated occurrence. It has been the story of his life; day after day he has experienced the indifference of others:

> For I have known them all already, known them all,
> Have known the evenings, mornings, afternoons,
> I have measured out my life with coffee spoons.

And the inaction of Alfred Prufrock is linked to his rock-bottom self-esteem. He is just a distant camp-follower on life's train and is all too aware of his inadequacies:

> No! I am not Prince Hamlet, nor was meant to be;
> Am an attendant lord, one that will do
> To swell a progress, start a scene or two,
> Advise the prince; no doubt, an easy tool,
> Deferential, glad to be of use,
> Politic, cautious, and meticulous;
> Full of high sentence, but a bit obtuse
> At times, indeed, almost ridiculous –
> Almost, at times, the Fool.

So for much of the time he retreats into a fantasy world where he can vaguely feel at home, until he is brought back to reality:

> We have lingered in the chambers of the sea
> By sea-girls wreathed with seaweed red and brown
> Till human voices wake us, and we drown.

Prufrock equivalents surround us everywhere, not just in the obvious form of people with obsessional personalities who hold on to fixed ways of behaving when it is clear to everybody else that they are doing nothing but harm, but also in the people restricted by fears that any new enterprise is fraught with danger, nicely illustrated by Chesterton's couplet, 'always keep a-hold of nurse, for fear of finding something worse', and in many others locked into humdrum lives and settings which at one level they want to change but seem powerless to do so.

In nidotherapy people with the Prufrock syndrome sometimes appear enthusiastic to cooperate at first and provide bold environmental changes for the nidotherapist to work on, but when these are seen to be too ambitious there is much less enthusiasm for the lesser ones that are feasible. These blocks in treatment are a challenge to nidotherapy and there are several ways of dealing with them. These include going round the obstacles instead of trying to climb over them, demonstrating in small environmental tasks that change is possible and the evidence for this should persuade even the most hardened sceptic, and acting as a buttress and sounding board for the patient when the courage to attempt change has finally been harnessed.

So J. Alfred Prufrock in treatment would have to take a break from pointless tea parties where he is humiliated by his inadequacies, replacing them with activities where he would feel more at home and in which the restriction of etiquette would no longer cramp his style. So after 6 months of nidotherapy we might see him as a pillar of the local rambling club, chatting naturally to an adoring audience of walkers as they brave the blustery winds of a 10 mile walk, knowing that great conversation and bonhomie will continue in the warm pub at the end of the trail.

The last concern is time. As the story of Dr Cawley's therapeutic encounter with Janet Frame indicates (see the prologue), the 'luxury of time' is important if nidotherapy is to show its full effects. Of course, every form of treatment now has to have a time label affixed, with recommended numbers of sessions and their duration at least suggested if not always adhered to, but nidotherapy, like many other treatments, does not offer a quick fix. At the end of this book I describe how nidotherapy can be delivered relatively economically in four sessions, but this is almost a minimum and if it is going to work at all much needs much to be done in the time between meetings with the therapist.

The prerequisites discussed here are summarised in Box 2.1. They can all be evaluated and decisions made in advance of a full assessment, but it is clear that a preliminary skirmish with the central issues is necessary before a patient is taken on.

Box 2.1   Requirements in advance of assessment for nidotherapy

- Before nidotherapy is considered all active treatments have finished their period of assessment.
- Mental state disorder is presumed to be chronic and persisting.
- Patient is supportive of the nidotherapy approach and consents to its use.
- Long-term nidotherapy input is feasible.

Prevent and predict

It should be appreciated by this stage that nidotherapy involves much more than listing a set of environmental requirements and then attempting to achieve them. People are complex – those with significant mental illness often much more complex than most – and amidst the ferment and torment of raging psychopathology the idea of planned environmental change is a distant fantasy. By getting a foothold in this chaos the therapist can often become the only acceptable guide to change. If the task is done well it becomes possible for the therapist to prevent the patient falling into further abysses of misfit and gives the marvellous bonus of predicting what might happen if certain changes were to take place. This can be checked to some extent retrospectively by looking through past records to see whether the therapist's predictions hold up.

To take one common example, the desire for autonomy, the most common theme in our nidotherapy assessments in those with severe mental illness, is understandable but it is not an all-or-none state. Its degree has to be balanced, and a good understanding of someone's level of personal organisation and ability to plan their lives can help to decide what level of autonomy is possible. Unfortunately in standard practice this process is far too often determined by trial and error. In an attempt to accede to the patient's wishes there is a gradual process of conferring increasing levels of independence to a point at which this has clearly failed. This commonly leads to a readmission to hospital and then the process, like a complicated version of the game of snakes and ladders, starts all over again. This expensive and demoralising tale is told over and over again in community mental health teams. The good nidotherapist should know at what point it is wise to say 'no' to further degrees of independence, and if the patient is fully in tune with the thinking behind this, they will also agree and not push the limits beyond which they should not go.

Exercise 2.1

A person with a diagnosis of persistent complaints about noise has been diagnosed sometimes with a delusional disorder and sometimes with schizophrenia. He has had repeated changes of housing over many years because in all of the placements he has been given he has been bothered by excessive noise. His complaints vary from heavy traffic noise outside in the street, whistling noises in the night, banging of ceilings and floors at unsocial times of the day and night, and high-pitched humming noises. The reasons why some health professionals feel he has schizophrenia is that these complaints seem to apply no matter where he is placed, and all attempts to satisfy his concerns appear to fail. He also gets very paranoid at times and feels that others are deliberately placing him in unsatisfactory accommodation as part of a campaign against him. He has identified certain individuals both within and outside the healthcare system who he is now convinced are trying to 'break him down' and get him admitted permanently to a mental institution. When challenged about this he becomes very angry and has been arrested for assault on more than one occasion but never charged. Treatment with antipsychotic drugs has been tried in a desultory way but no obvious benefits have been noticed.

Questions:

1   Is this patient suitable for referral for nidotherapy?
2   What information is needed before nidotherapy can be started?
3   What would be the essential elements that would need to be considered before taking him on for care?

CHAPTER 3

Environmental analysis

Environmental analysis has the potential to be confusing, because when interpreted too literally it can become an exercise similar to town planning. The intention is not to construct an ideal environmental set in which every need is accommodated, but to examine how things are now, how they could be changed and what would be the advantages and disadvantages of each change. There are two approaches to this task, the first being so much easier than the second.

Systematic arrangement and analysis of needs

This approach is used when the person concerned has a clear notion of what he or she wants and can weigh up the relative advantages created by success in achieving each of them. It can also be used by those who wish to carry out a nidotherapy assessment on themselves. This is much easier in the absence of significant current mental disorder, so that decisions can be made without any fear that the process will be handicapped by errors in judgement or subsequent changes of mind. The process is relatively simple. Every aspect of the environment is examined systematically and carefully and possible changes also examined for their positive and negative attributes. At the end of the analysis a set of agreed changes is decided, and the patient and nidotherapist move on together to the next stage of implementation.

Here is an example for illustration. Martinas is a middle-aged man who is mildly and chronically depressed. He comes from a central European country and has never felt completely at home since moving to the London area. He is married and his wife, who speaks very little English, is very dependent on him and now makes very few decisions herself, apart from those concerning her son, who is about to go to university in another part of the country. As he will be leaving home, the rest of the family are now thinking about moving to a smaller property, but Martinas has no energy for the necessary transactions in moving house and is becoming increasingly stuck in his ways. He realises it is not wise to do nothing but attempts to improve his depression by antidepressant therapy have all conspicuously failed and as he finds it an effort to talk about his symptoms and feelings in English he is not keen on trying most psychological therapies. Although he and his wife seem to be a devoted couple to outsiders, they have bitter arguments when on their own together and these make Martinas even more demoralised. He is therefore referred for nidotherapy and after assessment satisfies the criteria for this intervention (criteria as already discussed in chapter 2, pp. 14–17). When the assessment has been completed it is clear that Martinas is not severely depressed. True, he is demoralised and lacking in confidence, but he can feel much better when he meets friends from his own country and joins in celebrations of national events and anniversaries. He realises very early in treatment that the environment has a lot to do with how he feels. The nidotherapist sits down with him and produces three lists of possible environmental changes in the physical, social and personal environments that might have some value, and each is discussed in an open and collaborative way with new subjects introduced by either therapist or patient as needed.

Environmental analysis (Table 3.1; for tables please see the end of this chapter) identifies clearly that Martinas wants to move house and that there are few advantages in staying where he is. Congestion and noise pollution are both high and his current house is too large for his liking. But this alone is not a disaster. There is more than the physical environment to consider; the people and other social influences in the vicinity can have a major effect on personal preferences and attitudes (Table 3.2).

The last part of the environmental analysis is the need to explore the personal environment. Separating those aspects of the environment that are personal from those that are direct symptoms of mental illness is far from easy and there is bound to be some overlap. Nevertheless, this aspect of the environmental analysis is still important, as perceptions of the surroundings may be mistakenly attributed to mental state even when they are quite real and plain to see. Indeed, one of the strong reasons for getting out and about in the assessment for nidotherapy is to avoid the luxury of supposition and faulty assumption that what makes sense is automatically true (see Case study 9.3, pp. 77–79, for a good example). In Martinas' case there are clearly some personal environmental conclusions that could be accentuated by depressed mood (Table 3.3) but certainly not explained entirely by it.

The three parts of the environmental analysis are then brought together in making a summary that will enable environmental targets to be set in the next stage of nidotherapy. As the process to date has been a fully collaborative one, the summary also needs to be done together. For Martinas the full environmental analysis (Tables 3.1–3.3) might read:

> Martinas feels trapped in a lifestyle that he recognises to be unsatisfactory but one that he feels powerless to influence. He has a regular job and a settled family life but this lacks variety and he is under constant strain. His relationship with his wife is unsatisfactory and, although he does not use this word, he finds her a burden and wishes she could get a more independent life. He realises to some extent what he is missing when he meets his friends.

Although this happens all too seldom, he enjoys their company very much and his spirits lift whenever he is with them. His daily existence lacks any positive stimulation and there is very little to look forward to. Yet, despite all this, he recognises that a resolution of the problem is not impossible – a move to a different house could be one part of this, but he has no energy to initiate this and fears it will turn out to be a disaster.

This analysis is not especially profound or overflowing with telling insights, but it is a useful corrective to misperceptions that may be common in the analysis of psychological and pharmacological treatments. The depressed patient looks at life, according to one of my former teachers, John Pollitt, in a distorted way because of a physiological 'functional shift' (1960) and sees it through 'blue-coloured rather than rose-coloured spectacles' so that everything that happens is tinged with gloom. So, according to the treatment manual, the depressed perceptions of the environment do not reflect reality; rather than engage in changing the environment it is better to change the depression either through drug treatment (e.g. antidepressants) or psychological approaches such as cognitive–behavioural therapy (i.e. that address the 'distorted cognitions' that misinterpret the environment). But wait a minute. Martinas is in a rut – his life is going nowhere, his cherished son is about to leave home and only his wife will be there when he comes home in the evenings and she makes too many demands on him. Is all this a consequence of depression? I leave it for the reader to decide.

The conclusion I hope you will come to is that Martinas' environmental concerns are not entirely connected to his depressive illness, if indeed he has one, but are an important contributory factor that is worthwhile addressing. The attention paid to each of the elements in the analysis helps to construct a picture that is genuinely systematic and based on personal evidence, and could also be used as a springboard for action. Ever since I was a medical student I have been constantly warned never to allow people who are significantly depressed to make major decisions about their lives that could have long-term impact, on the grounds that when they are better they will regret what they have done and would never have gone ahead 'if they had been their normal selves'. Nidotherapy is the antithesis of this attitude but, as emphasised in chapter 2, the environmental analysis needs to be done at a time when mental difficulties have become chronic and are in some sort of equilibrium, and this often takes place when established treatments have failed or have achieved all that they are going to do.

Exploratory environmental analysis

The second form of environmental analysis may appear deceptively simple, but in fact it is not. In most of our work with chronic and severe mental illness it is difficult to get into an open and collaborative discussion of environmental needs. In our work with this group of patients they demand that health professionals stop interfering with their lives and the initial aims of nidotherapy may be focused, to the exclusion of other issues, on this particular goal. This leads to a uni-dimensional approach and an unsatisfactory outcome. Thus in addressing the nidotherapy needs of a patient in a restricted forensic environment (Spencer *et al*, 2009) it was not surprising in the qualitative analysis that the patient, 'whose primary goal was to achieve total freedom from restrictions', was disappointed as his goals were persistently thwarted. There may also be a surprising degree of ignorance about the range of environmental changes that may be available. The child who spends his life in a garret abused by both his parents has no idea what constitutes good care, and the lives of many with severe mental illness and personality problems, studded with adversity and deprivation from birth onwards, have often offered so little in the way of positive environments that these become to be seen as cartoon representations existing only in fairy stories. 'I want a house by the sea with my friends close by and a sandy beach where I can go for a swim every morning', said one of our patients when asked by her therapist what environment she would choose if she had the choice.

Sometimes the environmental wishes are negative rather than positive. Several of those we have seen in nidotherapy with antisocial personality and behavioural problems have embraced the idea of nidotherapy because they wish to stay out of prison, and many others just want all coercion to be removed from their lives, without having a clear alternative in mind. These are powerful motivating forces that can enable environmental analysis to proceed but in such cases it is often difficult to get a coherent strategy to move forward. Here the nidotherapist has to be inventive, to guide the patient towards a positive change that does fit in with their wishes and that can be tested out. Sometimes there is resistance even here; in what can be called the 'martyred bride syndrome' patients can become comfortably attached to the notion that all their problems can be attributed to forcible attachment to a treatment programme, lifestyle, accommodation arrangements or other settings that are against their real wishes. 'I know I said I wanted to be anywhere but hospital but I wasn't expecting to be put…', goes the refrain. Where the patient prolongs the martyr role is in claiming that there is nothing that they personally can do to change because an external authority or 'the system' is to blame for their predicament. This can become quite a comfortable position to hold because it avoids taking any personal responsibility for your future. 'You have put me in this awful situation, it is your job to get me out of it' has a satisfactory finality to it. When someone tries to prise open the lock and find a way forward that involves the patient taking at least some responsibility for what happens, as all nidotherapy should, then there can be resistance with obstacles being put up to every suggestion made for improvement. In these cases it is not possible to get a clear environmental analysis and possible nidopathway until later in the treatment. It is during this phase that the therapist will get a better notion of the likely duration of nidotherapy and the pace at which it should be moving and this should be taken notice of in supervision (see chapter 6).

Table 3.1   Environmental analysis – the physical environment of Martinas

Environmental area: physical environment	Need to change, Y/N	Nature of change (targets)	Priority
Accommodation	Y	Needs to move to a smaller house with less personal strain	High
Noise	Y	Present house is close to a flight path and the aircraft noise disturbs the family in the morning	Moderate
Pollution	N	Not especially concerned about pollution as he used to live next to a chemical factory in his native country	Low
Furniture	N	Attached to much of his furniture which was made in his native country and does not want to dispose of any of it	Low
Appliances (specify)	N	No problems	Low
Services (gas, electricity, heating)	N	No problems	Low
Carpets	N	No problems	Low
Curtains and fittings	N	No problems	Low
Cleanliness of area	N	No problems	Low
Transport links	Y	Where he lives the roads are very congested and public transport is poor, so he feels compelled to use his car in spite of wanting to be a 'good citizen' and reduce his 'carbon footprint'	Low
Temperature	N	No problems – the extra warmth in high summer does not bother him	Low
Humidity (dampness)	N	No problems	Low
Air quality	N	No problems noticed	Low
Light	N	No problems	Low

Table 3.2 Environmental analysis – the social environment of Martinas

Environmental area: social environment	Need to change, Y/N	Nature of change (targets)	Priority
Wife	Y	Would like his wife to be less dependent on him and to have more friends	High
Son	Y	Very fond of his son, likes his company, they have similar interests and get on very well; worries greatly how he will feel when his son leaves home	High
Neighbours	Y	Very little contact with neighbours living close by; thinks there is some prejudice against his family because they are not English; another reason for wanting to move	High
Friends	N	Would like to be closer to friends, most of whom come from his native country, but they live some distance away	Moderate
Privacy	N	No problems noticed	Low
Other family members	N	Although they all live some distance away, they get on very well together when meetings can be arranged	Low
Other people	Y	Most of the people in the area come from an older generation and ignore Martinas and his family	Moderate
Problems with authority figures (police, psychiatrists, council staff)	N	Martinas is a 'good citizen' and has no problems with authority figures and, if anything, may be too anxious to please them all	Low

Table 3.3   Environmental analysis – the personal environment of Martinas

Environmental area: personal environment	Need to change, Y/N	Nature of change (targets)	Priority
Feeling unsupported	Y	Everyone seems to depend on Martinas; he has no one to turn to for support	High
Feelings of oppression	Y	Feels surrounded by pressures bearing down on him continuously with no relief at any time	High
Social isolation	Y	On most days he meets only his wife and work colleagues and everything is predictable and uninteresting	Moderate
Lack of spare time	N	Has spare time but no interest in using it positively	Low

Exercise 3.1.

Dwain is a young man who has had several short admissions to hospital with 'brief psychotic episodes'. The exact nature of these episodes is far from clear: he makes frequent references to the 'the devil' and 'the force' when brought into hospital but cannot remember much about these on the following day. Enquiry reveals that on almost all of these occasions he admits to taking cocaine, ecstasy or cannabis – he cannot always remember which – and all these substances have been found in his urine at different times. When assessed for nidotherapy he has no clear aims in life and so it is difficult to assess his environmental needs. When asked about his future he replies 'Future? I don't care about anything after tomorrow – and that's not nearly as important as today'. Nidotherapy is the only treatment in town for Dwain, as he shows no interest in changing his drug use.

Questions:

1   How would you go about analysing Dwain's environmental needs in the light of his indifference to the environment?
2   What degree of cooperation would you need from Dwain before you attempted to carry out a nidotherapy plan?

CHAPTER 4

Reaching an agreement for environmental targets

Once the agreements for environmental change have been made in a formal manner using the tables described in chapter 3, or in an informal unwritten way which is probably more common, there needs to be a plan to implement those changes that are considered most important. This involves identifying the core environmental needs that are likely to influence many of the others if they are satisfied. This is one of the difficult parts of nidotherapy – it is not too difficult to get a list of apparent needs that are desired with greater or lesser enthusiasm, but identifying which are the core ones if someone has dozens is not an easy task. Thus a woman with constant need for support and encouragement may list a great number of individual needs such as contact with members of her family, regular meetings, being accompanied to shops and other places, holidays together, support when dealing with official matters, and the general needs for company. These cannot all be met as it would involve many people who have no particular desire to be involved regularly, providing support around the clock or at times to suit the individual rather than themselves, and there could be danger that they will repeatedly come into conflict with each other by making different arrangements. Together with the patient, the nidotherapist has to distil these needs into a practical and feasible way of providing the support that is needed and, once identified, this has to be confirmed with the individuals concerned to ensure that it is both feasible and viable in the longer term.

Often there may be considerable doubt about the best way of achieving these needs and in such cases it is often reasonable to test out suggestions before deciding on the best way forward.

Environmental tests

Environmental testing is similar to behavioural interventions in cognitive and behaviour therapy except that it is the environment being tested more than the patient's attitudes or behaviour directly. The essential elements involved in the environmental test are listed in Box 4.1. Although environmental change covers many elements, it is best to pick on a highly

---

Box 4.1   Principles of the environmental test

- Specificity: Test out one environmental change at a time wherever possible.
- Commonality: Ensure that the environment being tested covers a wide range of needs identified by the patient.
- Capability: The test is judged to be within the bounds of feasibility and capability of the patient to perform.
- Repeatability: The test is able to be repeated many times if necessary.

---

specific environmental change when testing out whether something is suitable rather than combining several elements and being unaware which is being addressed and which is being omitted. For example, it is extremely common for psychiatric patients who have been in hospital to have a period of leave at home before finally being discharged. In normal circumstances the exact nature of this leave, precisely when it would take place, who would be staying in the property at the same time as the patient, what support services would be available, and how the patient is planning to spend his or her time, are all possible questions that could be addressed but generally are left unsaid and unmeasured. In the case of nidotherapy a much tighter approach is necessary to answer a specific question. Thus for the patient involved who could not tolerate leaving hospital and felt nervous at home, it was necessary to specify a precise period of leave, who would be present at different times, and how the test would be monitored. This may seem obvious, but all too often such arrangements are largely left to the patient to decide what he or she would do, as outside hospital patients are free to do what they like. This is reasonable at one level, but in testing the environment it is always helpful to have a much more specific idea of what exactly is being tested and why.

Commonality refers to the ability to generalise from the environmental test. It is perfectly possible to test out a highly specific environmental change (e.g. having an alarm clock to wake you up in the morning so you can attend for your regular appointments), but there is little point in identifying such a test if it is so highly specific that its only function is to wake you up in the morning. If early rising is considered to be one of the major environmental needs, then the provision of an alarm clock may indeed be sufficiently specific and general, but it would be wise to have this backed up by other ways of ensuring an early start to the day.

There is no point in picking an environmental task that is either unfeasible or beyond the ability of the person to carry out. To extend the example mentioned earlier, it might be considered unreasonable to arrange for the patient needing support to get on a bus every day at 10 am for day hospital treatment in a trial period after discharge. This is particularly likely to fail if there are elements of agoraphobia or other avoidant behaviour as a consequence of the psychiatric problem. In this instance the activity required is really part of behaviour therapy rather than nidotherapy – the patient is being asked to move to a different environmental setting for support and care rather than having the setting altered directly at home.

A good environmental test needs to be repeatable. The opportunity for our dependent patient to fly 4000 miles to stay with his or her daughter in Canada is not a particularly good environmental test; it clearly is important but needs to be linked to other forms of testing that can be repeated if necessary and refined.

Degree of control

Collaboration is one of the fundamental principles of nidotherapy but sometimes this collaboration is more passive than is generally desirable. This particularly applies to many of those with chronic severe mental illness and personality disorder who have failed repeatedly to make progress during the course of treatment and who may have specific deficits with regard to motivation that have handicapped them throughout attempted rehabilitation. For those with less severe forms of mental illness who are able to take control of their lives it is relatively easy for a nidotherapist to set forth a number of possibilities with regard to improving the environment and for the individual concerned to decide which is important and should take priority and which should be relegated to another day. For those in whom the discussion of the environment rapidly moves in polysyllables to monosyllables a much greater degree of control has to be exercised by the therapist. In doing this it is very important to avoid the perils of paternalism. 'It seems to me that you should …' can easily become 'I have decided that you ought to do x because this is in your best interests'. Sometimes it may appear that the latter is indeed being carried out because there appears on the surface to be no ownership of the decisions made by the patient. Many people with the Prufrock syndrome will also be unwilling to commit themselves because of the fear of failure and long-term procrastination. However, the early stages of nidotherapy should have established fairly clearly what the patient wants to achieve with regard to environmental change. For a variety of reasons there may be many blocks to enable this change to take place and it is up to the therapist to try and overcome these as much as possible, and one of these blocks is the indifference of the patient.

Sometimes the opposite scenario may exist. The patient may feel extremely strongly that the only way forward is an environmental change that is felt by everybody else to be less than desirable and possibly full of risk. Here again the essential task is to be collaborative. For example, one of our patients with an intractable serious illness was particularly annoyed to have a psychotic diagnosis because, in his view, no matter what others might say, this represented complete separation between him and normal society. He battled at first against the diagnosis, one of the schizophrenia group, and eventually, when he agreed that he had such a condition that did make him different from other people, he came to the view that the only way in which he could be accepted in society again was to get married and have children. He told us this in the context of meeting another patient with significant mental illness and there was extreme uncertainty as to whether such a relationship would survive. Eventually, after much discussion in which the patient's trenchant views were expressed repeatedly and listened to, the team agreed to his marriage (they would have been powerless to prevent it but they gave it the seal of approval), and a year later he was the proud father of a baby daughter. Although in the long term the relationship was unable to be maintained, the childcare arrangements went well and, with paternity, a lot of the patient's worries about social exclusion were laid to rest. More importantly, he remained extremely fond of his daughter.

In discussing these issues the centrality of the relationship developed between nidotherapist and patient is clearly significant. Often the environmental changes discussed represent major personal decisions in a patient's life, and if they are to share this with the nidotherapist, a good relationship needs to be established in advance. A nidotherapist almost becomes a member of the patient's intimate family. All too often, such intimate relationships are lacking in those with severe mental illness and there is always the mix of danger and advantage that the nidotherapist may act as a substitute for these past omissions.

Boundaries for the nidotherapist

In attempting to tease out important environmental changes that will be fundamental to the patient's progress, the nidotherapist may be dragged hither and thither and appear to become what colleagues would describe as 'over-involved'. This may be particularly likely if the patient is being seen in their home environment and in other similar settings that are much more personal than a clinic or hospital. For that reason, establishing the boundaries in the therapist's relationship with the patient is crucial (Box 4.2).

Collaboration with the patient in nidotherapy does not mean that the nidotherapist should blindly follow wherever the patient wishes to go. At the same time it does involve a degree of following that goes beyond that in

---

Box 4.2   Setting the boundaries in nidotherapy

- Observation: Be aware of cues disclosed by the patient or observed by others that may indicate a more personal nature to the relationship.
- Past history: Check on previous risk assessments where past risky behaviour might be repeated.
- Prudence: Do not do in nidotherapy what you would not do in ordinary life.

ordinary practice. The conventional metaphor in such instances is a positive one. 'Going the extra mile' for a patient is considered to be an admirable attribute. It shows you care and, more particularly, it shows the patient that you care. So if you do something to help an environmental problem (the simplest one is paying for something that is needed and for which the patient does not have the money available to make payment themselves), then this goes beyond the ordinary boundary of clinical practice. The important point is that when these boundaries are crossed, they are clearly noted and accommodated accordingly. So if money is being spent by the therapist on something the patient should be able to afford, then the boundary can be reclaimed by the patient paying back the money later. Alternatively, if it is not appropriate for the patient to pay back the money, compensation has to be obtained from another source.

Although this is a simple example, it also applies to a wide range of other activities in nidotherapy. If the nidotherapist goes out of their way to see a patient in a setting that is preferred and familiar to the patient but unfamiliar to the therapist (e.g. a seedy public house), then it is reasonable for some sort of payback to be made by the patient as a consequence. So the therapist may well say 'I've gone out of my way to see you here this time, the next time I would like you to see me in my office because I want a bit more privacy and I think it is reasonable for you to make that extra effort now'.

The crossing of boundaries is also associated with the perception of increased risk. By entering too closely into the private world of the patient the assumption is often made that this is similar to trespassing on private property and running the risk of assault or prosecution as a consequence. In making a judgement about this the importance of trust, assumed to be developed in the early part of nidotherapy, is all important. The nidotherapist has to make a judgement in each area in which normal boundaries are being crossed as to whether there is sufficient danger for the intervention to be terminated or altered in some way (e.g. by having someone accompany the therapist in the setting). This is one of the important elements of supervision. An enthusiastic nidotherapist may be tempted to go further than is wise, but if a good case can be made for this then the supervisor may consider it appropriate. What should not be allowed to happen is for the banner of risk assessment to sweep all before it in an over-cautious approach that stifles progress in nidotherapy. In a qualitative analysis of nidotherapy in the setting of an assertive outreach team one of the strong positive consequences was that the team reviewed its attitude towards risk assessment as a direct result being made in nidotherapy (Spencer *et al*, 2009).

Nonetheless, it would be unfair to underplay the potential risks involved in nidotherapy, which involves developing a closer understanding of a patient's problems than would normally be expected, and in settings in which the therapist may feel somewhat vulnerable. In these circumstances it is wise to plan and anticipate what might happen in a particular setting and what limits need to be set on the nature and scope of the intervention. Thus, for example, if it is deemed necessary to give some information of a negative nature to a person who is impulsively aggressive, it may be wise to do so in a setting where there are others available in the vicinity who could help if any form of aggression is shown. All this comes under the general heading of prudence (Box 4.2), a quiet virtue that is often underplayed.

Duration of training for nidotherapy

It is not possible to train a nidotherapist in a lecture theatre or seminar room. A great deal of the necessary input has to result from *in vivo* experiences with patients being treated and the pace of progress depends greatly upon the previous experience of mental health and adaptability of the nidotherapist. This is discussed in Chapter 6 and wherever possible a supervisor is needed to cover the initial work of a novice nidotherapist. However, with the information in this book it is perfectly possible for someone with reasonable experience of mental health services to consider testing out nidotherapy, and if the setting is a well-supervised one (such as a care home where residents are regularly supervised), this may be particularly appropriate. Booster sessions of training for those who have already been working as nidotherapists may sometimes be needed, particularly when there is overlap between nidotherapy and other psychological approaches in which the patient is being treated directly (e.g. cognitive–behavioural therapy), or when a different patient population is being treated. It is perfectly appropriate to combine nidotherapy with other interventions but it should not be done without full awareness of when one crosses over to direct treatment of the patient who is leaving nidotherapy behind.

Exercise 4.1

A patient with a history of sex offending (harassing women in a pub when under the influence of alcohol) is taken on for nidotherapy to improve antisocial personality disorder functioning. His nidotherapist is female but experienced in dealing with people with personality disorder. In the course of nidotherapy it is recognised that the right sort of work is an important environmental need. When the patient is asked to attend for formal assessment of his ability to work he asked the nidotherapist to accompany him. This is considered appropriate as further information may be needed by the employment advisor. After the assessment the patient is deemed fit enough for work but only in certain areas that are free from children. Possibilities at the local job centre are identified and the patient again asks the nidotherapist to accompany him to the job centre to reinforce what he considers to be his safe behaviour but which he perceives needs back-up from the nidotherapist to ensure that a negative response is not automatic. The nidotherapist is not sure to what extent she needs to go to satisfy this particular environmental need.

What principles should be adopted in ensuring that the patient is given adequate support but important boundaries are not transgressed?

CHAPTER 5

Constructing and monitoring a nidopathway

The part of nidotherapy concerned with nidopathway has been given more prominence in other publications (Tyrer *et al*, 2003*a*; Tyrer & Bajaj, 2005), but our current thinking is that it is less important for most of the complex cases of people we see in treatment. This is not because it is unimportant, but it is one of the less complicated aspects of the treatment. If the groundwork has been done well, the nidopathway – a term that may appear unnecessary for what is basically a way forward – tends to go relatively smoothly, and if not, its correction is not difficult to make.

To illustrate this process we are going to describe what happened with somebody whose care followed a plan that was developed in the early stages of nidotherapy (Case study 5.1). This plan represented a radical departure from her previous treatment but because it had been worked out well in advance we had reasonable confidence that it was going to be at least reasonably successful.

Case study 5.1

Barbara was one of those patients who developed importance and fame – some might have called it notoriety – by being 'difficult'. Barrett (1996) has described this phenomenon in an anthropological study of a psychiatric hospital in which the staff and patients are seen as a cohesive group with clear but separate roles. The most difficult patients get a generalised label – usually their name or a derivative of it – that is immediately recognised by all the others in the group. So the question 'is this a Barbara problem?' in the hospital would conjure up an image of someone who dressed in the most bizarre of clothes, was innocently promiscuous without fully realising what she was doing, and who could not be allowed out of the hospital for fear she would wander off in a vague and irresponsible way and then require a search party to find her.

When she was not in hospital being treated for her schizophrenia, an exercise that stilted her activities a little but had no influence on their general style, she lived at home with her mother, who kept an eagle eye on her strange daughter

---

Here the early stages of nidotherapy have been condensed into one paragraph. A general issue of importance in developing a nidopathway is exemplified with Barbara at this point – that of novelty tinged with risk. For many who come to nidotherapy there is going to be a fundamental shift in the policy of care when the nidopathway is suggested. This is one of the reasons why it is given its slightly pompous name; it is a genuinely new strategy that contrasts strongly with what has gone before. It is a strategy that cannot be developed in a hurry, but rather is the culmination of the work that has been carried out in the quiet early stages of assessment.

The environmental analysis with Barbara suggested that:

- she wanted much more freedom in her life
- she indulged in risky behaviour partly as a reaction to the heavy restrictions that were normally placed on her activities
- she felt both the hospital and her mother were far too strict and never listened to her point of view
- she accepted she could not live on her own (a major achievement for the nidotherapist)
- she appreciated she needed guidance with her budgeting and living arrangements but could carry out most of the other tasks in life without supervision.

The tentative decision was therefore made by the nidotherapist, in this case a nurse, to suggest that a supervised placement with a family was the best option available to satisfy all these needs. If the right sort of place was found it would satisfy all the requirements of the environmental analysis by giving the 'long leash' type of supervision that could satisfy the concerns of the service and Barbara's wish for greater independence.

The nidopathway was now set. There was a clear element of risk, as Barbara's past history was a worrying one and led the proponents of good risk management to look for more restriction from the services rather than less in Barbara's life. A large part of this phase of the nidopathway was therefore a negotiating exercise. Would the team accept the nidotherapy analysis or not? In this instance it was not too difficult. Everybody else had

run out of ideas, so it was not too difficult to persuade those in authority to give this initiative a chance. But, naturally, with the increased risk it was necessary to give an assurance that she would be followed up very frequently once she left hospital.

The next stage was to match the intended nidopathway with the services on the ground. This often appears to be a hopeless task and far too often the next available option is taken rather than to wait until the right placement is available and then make changes to this to make an even better fit for the patient wherever this is possible. After a great deal of searching a family placement was found where Barbara felt comfortable, where the home routine was well-organised but low key, and which had good links with all the activities that Barbara wished to pursue. After a few trial days the agreement was signed and Barbara moved in.

Six years later Barbara is still living in the same setting and has had no admissions to hospital. She has a regular round of activities in her local neighbourhood but these are well-controlled and need no intervention from others. She seems happy and says she wants nothing extra in her life. In short, she is contented in her new nest.

Barbara's case illustrates a common issue in this stage of nidotherapy. There are very few environmental problems sufficiently serious to need nidotherapy that have an easy solution. So when a nidopathway is constructed it is rarely going to be implemented quickly. A pattern develops in which there are bursts of activity followed by the dead hand of bureaucratic silence, when everybody gets frustrated because no progress is being made. To reduce these as much as possible requires a great deal of effort away from the main stage, as it were, with back-room negotiations going on with a range of bodies and individuals who will have to agree things they do not normally agree to in order that the nidotherapy can continue. 'We are waiting for the housing association/local council/family/court/employer' – the list is almost endless – 'before we can move forward' is a frequent refrain in mental health services. At one level this appears to be irritating but for many it is an opportunity to sit back and have the enjoyment of doing nothing and passing the responsibility on to others in exactly the same way as the martyred bride syndrome described in chapter 3 (p. 27). These are the times when nidotherapists need to get their sleeves rolled up and tackle problems that are not insurmountable but do require a lot of effort and negotiation to overcome.

The monitoring of the nidopathway needs to be planned at the time it is set up. The key questions to decide are who should carry out the monitoring and how frequently it should be carried out? The ideal form of monitoring is one in which the person concerned takes a role as part of self-nidotherapy, but in the more difficult cases it needs to be either a professional or a group within the caring professions, who carries out this role as part of their other duties. The nidotherapist has a role too, but it is more usually placed at a secondary level. It is only when the standard monitoring suggests the nidopathway is going off course that alarm bells ring and the nidotherapist

is contacted to provide input. For this reason an important task at this stage of treatment is to train the individuals who will be carrying out the primary monitoring. This has to be done carefully and often delicately. The patient by this time should have developed an important personal relationship with the therapist and this may have involved sharing of sensitive information that is confidential. To avoid any tendency for the patient to feel abandoned or betrayed by the nidotherapist care has to be taken to transfer only that information that is relevant to the problem and to make it clear to the patient what is being shared and why.

Sometimes it may be considered wise for the nidotherapist to stay in touch with the patient by telephone during this period so that contact is not lost entirely. This is also a sensitive issue; some practitioners will allow their patients to telephone them on personal mobile telephones; others will insist that all contacts have to be made through formal channels and never disclose their numbers to anyone. The exact way of maintaining contact should fit in with the standard practice of the practitioner; what is important is for channels to be kept open between the nidotherapist, the patient and

Table 5.1   Range of actions in response to a failed nidopathway

Type of failure	General response	Specific examples
Planned environmental change is lost	Create new target as close as possible to the old one	Access to a chosen housing placement is denied, but an agreed alternative is found as soon as possible
New mental health problems intervene	The nidopathway is put 'on hold' until mental health is stabilised again	A patient develops acute depression and rejects the planned nidopathway as hopeless, insisting it has already failed
Failure of implementation by people involved in nidopathway	Rebolstering of faith in the nidopathway and replacement of personnel if necessary; no need to change the plan	The rules of a supervising agency prevent a chosen flexible plan of action to be implemented; after long negotiation with superiors these are changed
Patient's wishes change	Resetting of nidopathway, but only after careful evaluation of the depth of the wish to change and why	A patient who chooses to move to shared housing decides it is not working and asks for independent living arrangements; after finding that the problems are linked to one individual in the accommodation this decision is postponed
Targets achieved but recognised to be inadequate	A new nidopathway is constructed	With help a patient gets his flat redecorated and upgraded to a comfortable home but is then bored and lonely; new pathway to improve social contacts developed

the monitoring agency so that the nidopathway runs smoothly and any deviations from it are detected as soon as possible.

Many nidopathways, despite the best efforts of people to keep them on track, are going to fail. The response to these depends on the reason for failure (Table 5.1).

Failure to achieve the aims of the nidotherapy – to effect a better match with the environment – can be due to the disruption caused by the patient (change in mental state, change of environmental target), the staff involved in nidotherapy (external interference in the nidopathway), and by the nidopathway itself (a new perspective on environmental needs is developed). The ways of dealing with these are summarised in Table 5.1 and need very little explanation.

With ambitious nidotherapy targets the process of completion may take many years, long after personal therapeutic involvement in nidotherapy is completed. This does not matter; many of the intermediate points can be attained in a shorter time and continued striving for a further goal is the stuff of human endeavour; complacency is an enemy of good mental health.

Exercise 5.1

Margery is a woman of 25 with a mixed eating disorder of bulimia and anorexia. She has apparently responded to a treatment regimen mainly involving cognitive–behavioural therapy. Unfortunately, whenever she leaves the intensive contact she has at the hospital (she attends a day service four times a week) her problems return to some degree and are only reversed by increasing the frequency of day attendance again. In a nidotherapy assessment it became clear that the problems lying behind her eating disorder were closely linked to her parents and the reactivating of her symptoms was a consequence of living with her parents at home. She herself wishes to live away from her family but has never been on her own before and is lacking in confidence about what to do. She works part-time and has an income of just over £12000 a year, so has some resources to contribute to her housing.

Questions:

1 Formulate a nidopathway, including its planned length, which would enable Margery to live away from her family.
2 What should her family be told about this plan, and should it be the responsibility of the clinical team or the nidotherapist?
3 How frequently would the nidopathway be monitored and what should be the plan if there seems to be evidence of the symptoms and behaviour of her eating disorder returning?

CHAPTER 6

Supervision and training for nidotherapy

Nidotherapy is a form of management in development and its supervision and training are likely to change as it expands. The need for, and extent of, supervision will depend on the person concerned in treatment, the nature of the problem, and expected duration of nidotherapy.

Self-nidotherapy

It is perfectly possible for people reading this book to gather enough information to practise nidotherapy by themselves. With many treatments the adage 'a little learning is a dangerous thing' is a useful restraint on too much self-treatment, but as nidotherapy is only concerned with altering the environment in a planned and careful way it is very unlikely to lead to any significant adverse effects. I and my colleagues may have been uncritical in our own evaluation of the negative aspects of nidotherapy – this is a deficiency of all 'product champions' – but we have not been aware of anybody complaining that they have suffered because of exposure to this practice. In theory it is possible that a major environmental decision such as emigration to a distant country could be a consequence of nidotherapy, and if later regretted, would be difficult to reverse, but as the intention in all nidotherapy is to enable a person to generate a nidopathway in collaboration and to accept ownership of any plan, it would be important for such an important decision as this not to be taken in isolation.

The advantages of self-nidotherapy are that it can be conducted at the pace chosen by the patient, involves no conflict with others in its development, and can be constantly monitored and adjusted. It could be argued that a large number of people practise nidotherapy all the time in their daily lives – choice of occupation is an obvious example – and there are others who could practise it with benefit but who never have the nerve to make the environmental changes that are needed to improve their lives. It is perhaps most useful for those who are fully aware that they are not in tune with their environments and can half-understand what needs to be done about it, and who may find nidotherapy a help. These include many with the Prufrock syndrome discussed in chapter 2; these are not people who share their doubts and inadequacies readily with health professionals and often prefer to go it alone. Clearly in all these instances the patient acts as his or her own supervisor.

Co-nidotherapy

This term is not an ideal one but it refers to the many occasions when others close to the person needing nidotherapy may enable it to happen. The co-nidotherapists can be relatives, particularly spouses, close friends, employers, mentors and group representatives of all sorts. They can see first hand the need for environmental change and can help the person concerned to appreciate both the problems and likely solutions described elsewhere in this book. The need for co-nidotherapy is of especial relevance when there is conflict between two goals, one that involves the need for environmental change and the other that depends on maintaining the status quo even though it is doing damage. Co-nidotherapy is another intervention that many will come across in their own life. People who have long-standing goals that they seem unable to achieve on their own, in partnership can get to their goals and often beyond. The co-nidotherapist provides support, buttressing, motivation and resolve, and this without any need for training. In many ways this is the ideal form of nidotherapy assistance; it is sad that so many who come into the clinical frame for treatment have few people in their lives who even approach the foothills of this climb up to success.

Nidotherapy in mental health services

For reasons already discussed nidotherapy in mental health services is best carried out by a therapist detached from the clinical team. This is a potentially vulnerable position and the need for supervision of less experienced therapists becomes more important. Because nidotherapy takes place in a variety of different settings some of the standard ways of assessing whether the treatment is being given adequately (treatment fidelity) are not always appropriate. There is still the need to monitor what is happening in treatment sessions but this must not be carried out too rigidly, particularly with the complex problem where nidotherapy is being given indirectly, almost as it were in parentheses, with the main text expressed elsewhere. Nevertheless, however practised, nidotherapy involves a set of elements that are incorporated into a scale that the supervisor can rate (Nidotherapy Fidelity Scale, Table 6.1). Not all the individual subject items can be scored for some people, so the failure to complete part of the scale should not be regarded as a failure. The assessment of the nine sections is worth addressing in turn.

Table 6.1   The Nidotherapy Fidelity Scale[1]

Nidotherapy task	No evidence	Limited evidence	Substantial evidence
Score	**0**	**1**	**2**
General tasks			
Focusing on the environment rather than the patient's symptoms			
Separating functional gain from symptoms, behaviour or mental state			
Warm and friendly informality with few professional boundaries			
Ability to elicit the patient's views and wishes in a safe, understanding way			
Developing a trusting relationship with the patient's perspective as paramount			
Justifying the need for nidotherapy and its potential value			
Formulating a plan on how to deal with barriers to progress (such as disagreements, indecision, frustration, initial failure)			
Pacing the therapy at a rate appropriate for the problem			
Regular liaison with clinical teams and other service providers over the reason for and progress with nidotherapy			
Environmental analysis			
Exploring all the patient's current environments			
Selection of the best approach to defining the environmental changes both desired and needed			
Generation of a proper balance between the needs of the patient and those of others			
Formulating a nidopathway			
Getting a priority list of environmental needs			
Getting a plan agreed by all relevant parties			
Agreeing the priority order of environmental goals in terms of their timescale			
Implementation and monitoring of a nidopathway			
Setting explicit and discrete goals for monitoring progress			
Anticipating changes in targets wherever possible			
Maintaining the patient's agreement at every stage			
Giving a rationale for revising goals			
Joint negotiation of revised goals			
If goals are revised, gaining the patient's agreement with the revised goals			
Total scores			

1. Original scale (unpublished) prepared by Tom Sensky; subsequently modified after field experience

General nidotherapy assessment tasks

All the components of this section are involved with assessing the therapist's style and general approach throughout nidotherapy.

1. Focusing on the environment rather than the patient's symptoms

Most of the nidotherapists in our developmental work have not been therapists in mental health before coming to nidotherapy. This is seen as more of an advantage than disadvantage, as for many staff the pressure to treat or alleviate symptoms trumps all other requirements and can interfere with nidotherapy. The good nidotherapist acknowledges symptoms and behaviour as important, and can support the patient in appreciating the suffering they can cause. But, and here the treatment is quite different from other forms of practice, the therapist does not try to change them in any way unless this change is clearly linked to the planned nidotherapy. Many questions about symptoms can be deflected into 'environmental mode', so 'I don't know what to do with these feelings of depression that bother me all the time' can be deflected into 'I can understand how bad you must feel, but are there circumstances you have been in or other times recently when your depression has been somewhat better?'

2. Separating functional gain from symptoms, behaviour or mental state

This is a natural corollary to the previous section. Nidotherapy is about fitting the environment to the person, and when it has been achieved there has, by definition, to be a better level of function and general adjustment. Symptoms demand relief and removal and are very different from functioning, and even though they are naturally considered by patients to be more important than functioning (Crawford *et al*, 2008*b*), functioning is of probable equal importance generally, and probably more important in most of those coming for nidotherapy. It is also useful to emphasise to the patient the importance of general functioning if and when, as patients often will, they complain about the failure of the therapy to address their symptoms. 'I said at the beginning that I was not treating your symptoms', can be the reply, 'we planned on improving things in your life to make a better fit for you, and this is the way we hope you will feel better, not by treating your symptoms.'

3. Warm and friendly informality with few professional boundaries

It cannot be stressed too often that most of the people in mental health services who are involved in nidotherapy have already had a great deal of treatment and, possibly more importantly, a great number of therapists. To take one person from my own experience, a man who had attended an out-patient department at 6-monthly intervals for 15 years irritatingly told me that he had seen 35 doctors in that period, 30 of them being the junior doctors who had changed every 6 months so that each one was seeing him for the first time. 'It wouldn't have mattered,' he told me ruefully, 'but every single one of them had to go over my history again, so I felt I was just a teaching exercise for them'.

So for these people the nidotherapist will be viewed askance as yet another enthusiastic visitor who will briefly pass the time of day before riding off into the sunset, quite indifferent to what they have left behind. It is imperative that the nidotherapist has the ability and interest to concentrate and listen carefully to everything that concerns the patient in the first few contacts to set down the bedrock of collaboration and cooperation that will be essential later on. A therapist who comes back to supervision and says 'I don't like Mr X at all, but am determined to try and work with him' is not going to do especially well in nidotherapy, as the ability to get on the same wavelength as the patient is needed if the right environmental steer is to be provided.

Many are naturally concerned with the importance of maintaining professional boundaries with patients because of the risks attached. This has already been addressed in chapter 4 (pp. 34–36); the natural caution that needs to be employed when seeing people away from a familiar clinical environment should not prevent the interchange of equals when it comes to sharing views and opinions. So if a patient comments on how difficult it is to deal with a rebellious teenage son it is perfectly appropriate for the nidotherapist to join in with his or her experiences with the same problem, not just as an exercise in maintaining the flow of discussion but also to help in promoting the beginnings of an honest understanding, not a phoney effort at bonhomie that is suppressed as soon as it arouses a response.

4. Ability to elicit the patient's views and wishes in a safe, understanding way

A person who has failed to respond to treatment repeatedly, especially when it is evidence-based (i.e. the implication is that it is the patient, not the treatment, that has failed), or someone who has failed to recognise, rightly or wrongly, that a treatment of any sort is considered necessary for their problems, is not usually well disposed to disclose what they feel should be done in an open and gentle way. Their opposition to what has been tried already and what they feel is the right way to proceed may have been shouted from the roof tops but in monologues and cameo performances, not in conversation or quiet discussion. A new approach has to be developed in nidotherapy in which every single aspect of the patient's view of the world and their place in it has to be taken seriously and carefully, no matter how illogical and unreasonable it appears to be. In supervision the therapist's generosity and patience are very important attributes to detect.

5. Developing a trusting relationship with the patient's perspective as paramount

It is no use being able to elicit the patient's underlying aims and wishes without taking notice of them and giving them proper status. This is not easy, because some apparent wishes may appear capricious and not worthy of proper consideration. However, even the most inappropriate of aims can be used to make a useful gain. Take the following conversation with a young man of 25:

> Therapist: 'What would you really like to do when you leave hospital?'
>
> Patient: 'Set up and run a cannabis farm.'
>
> Therapist: 'I'm not sure if that's legal, but why would you want to do this?'
>
> Patient: 'Well, when I look at my life I know I'm only happy when I have cannabis, so I want it whenever I need it.'
>
> Therapist: 'Have you ever tried growing cannabis? I'm a gardener and I think it would be hard work.'
>
> Patient: 'Why's that?'
>
> Therapist: 'Cannabis grows in hot countries and needs a lot of light, so you would have to be able to have very careful temperature and light control each day or you would lose your crop. The plants would need very careful attention.'
>
> Patient: 'I'm not so sure about this now. Perhaps I'll just have some in the porch.'

Some people would regard this conversation as a pointless exercise. No one is going to approve the environment of a cannabis farm and so conversation about it is redundant. But it does serve a purpose. It gets the patient to think about the practicalities of growing cannabis and gives some understanding of the difficulties but, more importantly, it shows that the therapist is taking the patient seriously. The patient's views may be wrong-headed, unbalanced or just plain crazy, but each needs to be explored as though it was a serious, well thought out option. The respect the patient will build up for the therapist in this exercise will be very useful later on in therapy. Even if there is an element of game-playing in the patient's propositions, the very fact that they are taken seriously is an important jolt to the patient's understanding. 'This guy's a bit funny, but he's not just dismissing my ideas, so perhaps I ought to think about them a bit more carefully too', is the common response to this approach.

6. Justifying the need for nidotherapy and its potential value

Nidotherapy in some form or another has to be justified openly in treatment sessions. It can be talked about indirectly along the lines of 'We are looking at the best situation possible for you' and then describing each of the elements of the environment that when changed would define what is 'best', or directly by discussing the principles behind the treatment and why it is being chosen. This also needs to bring out the differences between attempts to change the environment in the past and what is being tried now, and how important it is to get the patient's views on each part of this process. At one level we are trying to get the patient to sign up to this approach and possibly be even enthused by it (but we must not expect too much and great enthusiasm is rare). Participation by the patient in the nidotherapy process is far from easy to achieve, but at some level it needs to be attained. Reminders about what it is and why it operates in the way it does, need to be made at least occasionally.

7. Formulating a plan on how to deal with barriers to progress

It is very rare for nidotherapy to proceed without disagreement. Indeed, it can almost be said that a course of treatment without any dissent between therapist and patient is an indication of a superficial, probably too superficial, form of the treatment. The simple fact is that those who recognise that their environments are not right go about changing them and usually do so quite effectively without ever feeling that they have taken part in a therapeutic exercise. Those who are referred for nidotherapy fall into three main groups. The first does not know what changes are going to be right for them and need a great deal of help in finding the right ones. They are bound to disagree with some of those suggested by the therapist at least once or twice in the course of treatment. The second group dogmatically insists they know exactly what they need and complain that everyone is stopping them from achieving that. It does not take much thought to realise that argument is just round the corner here. The third group seems to have a good idea what is needed but never seems to achieve any progress towards this. This group includes the 'martyred brides' (see chapter 3, pp. 27), who are gently wallowing in self-justified inactivity reinforced by blaming others, and others who are chasing the rainbow of environmental gain but never seem to get there, for reasons that are never entirely clear. They may be going too far too quickly, or may have unrealistic ideas of their abilities, or are just unlucky in having no allies or supporters. This group can get very frustrated and angry in treatment and will not withhold this from the nidotherapist.

8. Pacing the therapy at a rate appropriate for the problem

The rate at which a nidotherapy treatment plan is implemented is tremendously varied. Often progress seems to be very smooth but then comes to a series of stuttering stops before moving on again. This is because so much of nidotherapy is beyond the nidotherapist's control, and in this way it differs from many other psychological treatments. Inexperienced therapists are sometimes inclined to expect too much too soon. Indeed, one of the most consistent messages we have received from patients in nidotherapy has been the appreciation of the time spent in talking about problems that have too often been glossed over with other professionals. The 'marvellous luxury of time' noted by Janet Frame in her treatment with Dr Cawley is really not a luxury but a necessity in good nidotherapy.

So it is important for supervisors to try and set realistic timescales with nidotherapists. Sometimes these may be forced, as in the extreme position described in chapter 9, where the tightest plan is to introduce all of nidotherapy in only four sessions. In planning the pacing of nidotherapy both the direct contact with the patient and the indirect groundwork in developing environmental targets with others have to be taken into consideration, as indeed has the setting in which nidotherapy is taking place. Particularly in the early stages, when meetings can be taking place in settings chosen by the patient but which are quite unsuitable for intimate conversation and personal disclosure, it is important to allow for these potential difficulties. For this and other reasons, the recording of interviews to test fidelity is not always possible and is probably not the best way of assessing the fidelity of the treatment.

9. Regular liaison with clinical teams and other service providers over the reason for and progress with nidotherapy

One of the central components of nidotherapy mentioned several times in this book is the value of keeping the nidotherapist independent from the clinical teams who normally look after the patient. In a qualitative study of nidotherapy given to patients with antisocial personality disturbance – one of the most difficult but rewarding areas of nidotherapy – three of the eight negative themes in the analysis referred to the problems of liaison between the clinical team and nidotherapist (Spencer *et al*, 2009). This was most prominent with the treatment of in-patients. In the words of one of our nidotherapists, 'it was very difficult to plan anything for (this patient) because it would always be overridden by policy on the wards'. Even with the more flexible arrangement of community mental health teams it is often difficult to get the right balance between working in confidence with the patient and sharing information with the team, as Case study 6.1 indicates.

There is no easy answer to this problem, and it is very easy for frustrated therapists to blame each other when things go wrong. It is probably best to get agreement with the patient on how liaison will take place with the clinical team at the onset of nidotherapy to avoid problems like this from developing.

Competence and achievement of the general tasks in nidotherapy continue to develop over the course of treatment. Using the scoring system of the Nidotherapy Scale (see Table 6.1, p. 44) a supervisor should expect at least a total score of 10 in the General Section early in treatment, rising to at least 14 by the end.

> **Case study 6.1**
>
> A woman with a complex mix of personality problems comprising severe per-
> sonality disorder was very reluctant to engage with her clinical team because
> she blamed them for many of her environmental difficulties. When she saw her
> nidotherapist she emphasized the need to keep their conversations secret. Subse-
> quently she refused to see the clinical team at all and only saw the nidotherapist. It
> was felt by the nidotherapist that continued liaison should be maintained with the
> clinical team and so this continued intermittently. This unfortunately was picked up
> by the patient and so the nidotherapist too was sacked. The problem was resolved
> eventually but not after considerable troubles in the interim, and the consequence
> was that the patient ended up with a single therapist.

Other sections of the Nidotherapy Fidelity Scale

The remainder of the Nidotherapy Scale is specifically linked to the stages
of nidotherapy that do not all need to be considered in supervision.

Environmental analysis

In the environmental analysis all aspects of the environment need to be
addressed, even if only one or two are deemed to be important. This is
because many hidden needs can be identified in a full analysis but, perhaps
more importantly, the exercise of going through each area helps to get a
better understanding of all aspects of the patient's functioning and helps
the advocacy role of nidotherapy. So the nidotherapist needs to explore
all the patient's current environments over the course of this part of
nidotherapy. The decision has to be made early in the course as to whether
the assessment is done in an open and transparent way with the patient
(as with Martinas, chapter 3) or whether it is preferable to do it indirectly
because the patient does not have the necessary organisational skills, is too
suspicious of what looks like an 'official' approach to the analysis, or is too
focused on one aspect of the environment to the exclusion of all others.
Once the wishes of the patient become known the next part of this analysis
is to achieve a balance between these and those of both the immediate
neighbours and others close to the patient and wider society. This has to be
handled gently at times, because it is very easy for a patient to feel fobbed
off by a therapist who can be accused of having made their mind up already
and steamrollering a plan that has very little true collaboration incorporated
within it.

Formulating a nidopathway

If the environmental analysis has gone well it should be possible to formulate
a nidopathway without too much difficulty. There may be argument about
linking the main needs to the pathway, as the more practical pathways are

often considered of secondary importance by the patient. Getting the plan agreed by everybody can also be a delicate task and requires a separate set of skills. A lone nidotherapist is not in the best position to carry the day against a powerful lobby of clinicians and managers who disagree and can be intimidated into adopting a revised pathway that may not be the one preferred by the patient or the nidotherapist. But compromise is of the essence here, and the nidotherapist may need the help of the supervisor to come to the best possible arrangement that can be embraced by all as one in which each practitioner has made a unique contribution.

After the plan has been agreed it is necessary to have at least some idea of the timescale for the nidopathway, not least because patients sometimes expect more rapid results than professionals do. In doing this it is wise to be more pessimistic than optimistic so that subsequent attainment of targets is greeted with more enthusiasm.

Implementation and monitoring of a nidopathway

This is the very practical part of supervision. A nidopathway has been created and agreed but many changes can intervene before it can be completed. This can be distorted by change in the timescale, adjustments to the preferred targets, and a change in the attitude of the patient. It is best to anticipate as much as possible some of the more likely changes that are not part of the nidopathway. This does not mean that every possible eventuality has to be discussed but it is usually clear where there is uncertainty in the pathway. 'What would you think is the best thing to do if…?' is a good question to put to all people involved in developing and monitoring the course of treatment. In mental health assessments this comes under the headings of 'crisis management' and 'actions to be taken at signs of relapse'. In the same way problems with the nidopathway can also be anticipated and corrections made.

The scale is best scored at the end of nidotherapy, when a score of 14 on the Nidotherapy Fidelity Scale indicates an acceptable level of performance. A nidopathway may not be completed for several reasons that are entirely beyond the control of the nidotherapist. This does not prevent a high score being given on the Scale if all the elements have been addressed properly.

Supervision of nidotherapy is best carried out by someone who is experienced in the treatment, but at present nidotherapists are few in number. We currently organise an Annual Nidotherapy Conference every year and training sessions take place there, but it is really only when therapy is in full flow in a service that all the important issues come into focus. There is also a case for the supervisor being a senior member of another clinical team, as the issues about professional boundaries, the best form of liaison with clinical teams, and action to be taken at times of disruption to the nidopathway can often be answered most effectively by a senior professional within the existing service.

CHAPTER 7

What are the qualities of a good nidotherapist?

Nidotherapy is not for the faint-hearted, but neither is it for the exceptionally sophisticated of therapists. It also cannot be learnt easily as a technique in the same way that some psychological therapies can. Of course, there are technological aspects of the treatment, and these are dealt with elsewhere in this book. This chapter is concerned with natural qualities that have become part of a therapist's repertoire in ordinary life. There are three general requirements without which little progress is likely to be made no matter how much formal training is received. The first is openness. In studies of normal personality patterns openness is one of the so-called 'big five' personality factors (Costa & McCrae, 1992). It describes the ability to be open to new experiences, willing to step outside one's own immediate setting and its requirements, and willingness to accept the feelings of others as equally valid as your own. This is not the same as being gullible or naive, as although at times openness may lead to the person being manipulated to some extent, openness grounded in reality and linked to awareness of circumstances prevents too much uncritical acceptance.

The second requirement is achieving trust. This is particularly important with people with long-term mental health problems. Time after time conventional psychiatric input makes vague promises that are often poorly delivered. This is why one frequently gets complaints along the lines of 'You people are all the same. You come along full of promises, giving me hope that something's going to be done, and then in the end let me down, making all sorts of excuses as to why you failed. Is it surprising then that I don't trust you?' A central component of achieving trust is not to promise things that you cannot deliver. When demands are made early on in assessment it is much better to answer 'I don't know' than make empty assertions that you cannot back up or blanket refusals when you are unaware of the full situation. Trust is easier if it is completely reciprocated, but there are many occasions when the nidotherapist may feel that the patient cannot be trusted in many different respects. This does not obviate the need for everything possible to be done to engender trust in treatment.

Enabling skills is also an essential part of the style of the nidotherapist. This has to strike an important balance between passing on your own skills to the patient and putting these into action so that an element of imitation, or modelling, can take place. It is likely that success has evaded many of those requiring treatment, and training in ways of being successful is an important component of the treatment. This does not mean the therapist showing off skills that the patient will never be able to obtain, but when an appropriate time comes in treatment something that the patient finds difficult can be done by the therapist. One of the unfair assumptions about many people of reasonable intelligence who have chronic mental illness is that they have the ability to do everything that other people can do, particularly in faring for themselves in the essential necessities of life. Unfortunately mental illness leads to at least temporary incompetence and incompetence often breeds further incompetence that pursues a cycle of its own. Many of the skills to be taught to the patient are basic ones that the therapist may not feel are important, but if they are taught and demonstrated clearly to the patient it is amazing how valuable they can be.

My view, which can only be a preliminary one at this stage of learning, is that many people have the innate attributes to be good nidotherapists without fully realising they have this ability, and this is because they have curiosity, humility, charm, persuasiveness, persistence and patience, all of which are necessary in effective treatment (Box 7.1).

Curiosity (of a non-voyeuristic nature) is almost a prerequisite in nidotherapy. On the surface many of those who have persistent and recurring mental illness are unattractive and uninteresting to other people. The exceptions, of which a prominent example is Stephen Fry, the broadcaster, commentator and wit, and who also has bipolar disorder, are those who are able to maintain a good world view and have the ability to get over to others sympathetically how they are when they are unwell. (In Stephen Fry's case I suspect a little self-nidotherapy has gone into his strategy for dealing with it successfully without the need for formal psychiatric help.) One reason why those with chronic illness may seem 'uninteresting' is that prolonged suffering, whatever its form, tends to restrict a person's horizons greatly and the suffering created by it is very difficult to communicate without doing

---

Box 7.1 Essential elements that assist in nidotherapy

- Curiosity: a genuine interest in people and why they are the way they are
- Humility: recognition that other people's opinions and views may often be more relevant to them than your own opinions
- Charm: the ability to engage people in a positive way without being patronising, insincere or dominating
- Persuasiveness: the ability to get people to address matters that often they would prefer to avoid, embrace or discard with simple unthought options
- Persistence: the quality of continuing to try when all around have given up long ago
- Patience: the willingness to spend time with people when they need it even though it may seem to be unnecessary to everybody else

so in a way that seems harsh, one-sided and hypercritical of others. The curious go far beyond this point, and in nidotherapy come to understand why people behave and think the way they do because of the situations they find themselves in. So a common example is when others get frustrated and say of such a patient 'I can't understand why he/she does not get in touch with the council/go to the Citizen's Advice Bureau/arrange an appointment with the housing officer. He/she is quite capable of doing this and is not short on intelligence. What's stopping him/her?', and you suspect that none of the people who say this are all that interested in finding out the answer. As part of the first stage in nidotherapy a clear task will be to find out exactly why the person has such an engine of inaction and cannot do what appears blindingly obvious to others. You often have to dig deep to get the answer and curiosity helps enormously in doing this.

One of the problems of being trained well in any discipline is that it teaches you to take shortcuts in order to increase efficiency. So in mental health assessment the excellent and experienced consultant will often interrupt the patient in the mid-flow of a soliloquy and ask a question or make a decision that is clearly intended to shorten debate and move on. In nidotherapy this is not appropriate except in difficult and risky situations and it clearly perpetuates the belief that it is right to overrule the judgement of the patient as something that can be lightly disregarded as the product of an overheated brain. In assessing what people want and need in their environments all explanations should be considered and all have equal validity if they are deeply felt. So a humble nidotherapist is a good therapist and can genuinely say 'You have really taught me something' after a conversation with the most unproductive of respondents.

We noted earlier that nidotherapy is often chosen after all other therapies have been abandoned. Even though it is emphasised that the environment is the focus of attention rather than symptoms or behaviour, it is still often difficult to engage the patient in the treatment. By the time a condition has become persistent or relapsing a weary cynicism has crept into discussions about new forms of help, as though both therapist and patient are on probation after multiple offences and neither really believes anything is going to change. In this situation personal charm is an amazing ally. Even if the patient at first has absolutely no faith in what is being proposed, when they can be stimulated sufficiently at interviews to want to know more, have their beliefs challenged or curiosity aroused, or even just want to see the therapist again, then progress has been made. Often humour can be combined as an element of charm but this has to be handled sensitively if it is not to be regarded as mocking.

Although a nidotherapist in evaluating the environment is engaged on a voyage of discovery in largely uncharted territory, there is a constant requirement to bring the patient alongside as an active participant and collaborator. This is where persuasiveness comes in. If the patient sits as a passive spectator watching as the nidotherapist weaves a complex design of targets, end points and performance charts, this becomes a pointless exercise that means little and leaves the patient puzzled and frustrated. Just as the skills of a cognitive therapist enable the patient being treated to remain active in the engine room of therapy, so the skills of the nidotherapist ensure that the decisions made about the environmental changes are not just generated by the therapist and rubber-stamped by the patient, but are embraced as a joint enterprise which, in the last resort, is owned by the patient.

The nidotherapist also has to have the attribute of persistence. Nidotherapy can be extremely frustrating and sometimes demoralising if it is regarded as similar to other forms of treatment. Because, often unintentionally, an abnormal behaviour is repeated just because the environments in which it becomes manifest are also repeated, both therapist and patient, and others in the clinical team, can all say 'There you are, nothing is happening. He is just the same as ever. No progress has been made. Why are you wasting your time?'

Patience is this pressured age is an admirable virtue, and it is often needed in abundance in nidotherapy. Because horizons become so constricted in chronic forms of mental disability, preoccupations that seem unimportant to the therapist can become all-consuming to the patient and take up what appears to be needless time. But all time spent in nidotherapy can be used positively and it is useful to think of something that can almost be formulated as a golden rule: 'The less in touch I feel with the patient, the more likely I am to discover something useful in nidotherapy.'

Professional training for nidotherapy – who should administer it?

What professional training would be useful for those who wish to practise nidotherapy? The qualities described above are human qualities that are not exclusive to any single professional group. They can, and should, be shared across the board but, nevertheless, some training is much more relevant to nidotherapy than others.

Psychiatrists

Psychiatrists have a hard time becoming good nidotherapists. First, they are seen as agents of 'person change' rather than 'place change' and tend to be stereotyped in that role. They are also seen, at least for those with severe mental illness, as adverse environmental agents who deprive people of their liberty for no good reason and detain them in places where they suffer and are unhappy. They also have the tendency, often denied, to be paternalistic with their patients, deciding what is best without giving an opportunity for other options and possible compromise. Over the course of the years when I have been practising nidotherapy I have been accused of being taken for a ride by patients who unmercifully exploit me, being a sucker for punishment, deskilling the profession, laying myself open to accusations of malpractice, and just being plain stupid, as I should be 'keeping a proper lifestyle and staying in the hospital waiting for patients with schizophrenia'. So my advice to psychiatrists is to tread carefully before jumping in the nidotherapy pool. If you do take the plunge, remember that it may take some time before your colleagues come round to your way of thinking.

Social workers

Social workers, on the other hand, despite their active involvement in assessments under the Mental Health Act (together, in England, with many others who perform this role), can almost turn to nidotherapy as one of the theoretical underpinnings of their profession. In making assessments in a social work context the physical and social environment is always being considered as a priority. In making a mental health assessment the social worker is always exhorted to choose 'the least restrictive form of care', and acts almost as a citizen's advocate in this role. This is what a good nidotherapist should be doing all the time, and it is no coincidence that in our work the need that is craved above all others is the wish for autonomy – the ability to make one's own decisions in life without being interfered with, however benevolently, by others.

Clark (2000) has described the four core principles of social work, which he says are often misleadingly called values, as:

1   the worth and uniqueness of each individual
2   entitlement to justice
3   essentiality of community, and
4   the claim to freedom.

Nidotherapy, an enterprise that is determined to look at the world through the eyes of the patient, and so experiencing their feelings and hopes, is consistently trying to promote the worth and uniqueness of the individual, to represent them in a difficult world when sometimes all the dice seem to be stacked against them, and to promote independence wherever possible. Indeed, the promotion of independence within normal society, which is equivalent to Clark's 'essentiality of community', is one of the main gains of nidotherapy in practice. When added to standard care in an assertive outreach team, patients randomised to the additional nidotherapy spent much less time in hospital and were in less expensive community accommodation than those in ordinary assertive outreach care, so that for each patient given extra nidotherapy over £4000 was saved per year (Ranger *et al*, 2009).

Social workers can therefore justify 'the least restrictive' option not only on ethical grounds but on practical commercial ones. They are also very well placed to be nidotherapists as it is typical for them to be at least one step removed from the rest of the psychiatric clinical team with regard to its principles and practice. There tends to be a certain conflict between the social work and psychiatric professions because of their different traditions, and although this has its negative aspects, including a high rate of burnout and stress among social workers (Evans *et al*, 2006), the positive ones include the ability to act independently in an advocacy role with patients and at times represent them against the rest of the team. This is pure nidotherapy and should be celebrated for its diversity. The good social worker is also clearly based in the community, knows its values and expectations, and is often much more aware of the settings in which the average patient lives than many others in the mental health services.

Psychologists

Psychologists also have the potential to be good nidotherapists. They are excellent at establishing good working relationships with patients and working in a collaborative way. One snag is that they sometimes have a compulsion to treat, and in the course of nidotherapy may slip into this conflicting role and create problems for themselves and the patient. There is also a wish to complete therapy in a fixed number of sessions and although we have been drawn into this Procrustean trap in chapter 9, it is much better to allow much more flexibility in the nature and timing of nidotherapy than would normally be tolerated. But we acknowledge that there is a definite overlap between some psychological treatments and nidotherapy, particularly with cognitive and behaviour therapy.

Nurses

Nurses also have the ability to be good nidotherapists, particularly when attached to community teams, as they then become used to assessing people in a variety of settings and work in a multidisciplinary way. Those who are trained as graduates in other subjects before coming to nursing may be particularly suitable. One example is the mental health practitioner programme, which goes beyond traditional nursing training and scope by addressing all the psychiatric models (Tyrer & Steinberg, 2005) in their work. This allows easy collaboration with all front-line staff in multidisciplinary teams and can easily embrace nidotherapy as the epitomy of the social model in this scheme. This also includes aspects of clinical psychology and occupational therapy that reinforce their knowledge base and philosophy of practice (Brown *et al*, 2008). One possible problem that traditional nurses have when coming to nidotherapy is that the 'need to care' may sometimes supplant the 'need to reflect' on the settings and situations that will need to be changed in nidotherapy. But this can be changed – the important thing is not to try and match the two roles at the same time as this will interfere with assessment and management.

Housing support workers

Housing support workers and, indeed, housing officers in their administrative roles, see a great deal of mental illness and are good assessors of pathology (Marriott *et al*, 1993). They are often the unsung heroes and heroines in community mental health services, when they pop up out of nowhere and find a placement for somebody that no one had thought existed. But success should not always come suddenly like winning a lottery, and incorporating such housing experts into the nidotherapy structure is an excellent way of adding a systematic element to the placement of a patient. But these skills have often been honed over many years and can be generalised to much more than the single environmental issue of housing. A whole range of activities that used to be described as those of daily living (Marx *et al*, 1973) can involve skills and special knowledge that only the housing expert can access.

Occupational therapists

Occupational therapists can vie with social workers as occupying the place where nidotherapy should feel most at home. Although clearly nidotherapy takes the therapist into many areas where an occupational therapist would feel unfamiliar, the general principles of occupational therapy, to enable the patient to fulfil their own wishes and activities in their favoured environment, is just right for nidotherapy.

Despite these suggestions, in our own practice almost all the nidotherapists we have trained to date are 'outside the system', in that they had not been trained as professionals in any mental health service before they started their work in nidotherapy. Clearly, therefore, we would argue that a qualification in a mental health subject is not a necessity before entering the field of nidotherapy, and in some ways it is an advantage not to have the training of an alternative form of care interfering with the nidotherapy. The experimental psychologists call this 'proactive inhibition', the knowledge of earlier experience inhibiting the acquisition of new material. So it is perhaps no accident that our core of nidotherapists comprise a general physician with an interest in mental health, a research psychologist who has not been employed clinically, a medical student who may choose to be a psychiatrist in due course, and a doctor who started nidotherapy after basic training and only now is on course to become a fully qualified psychiatrist. But the nurses are also knocking at the door and are also improving their skills. We feel the eclectic mix of different disciplines has been an aid to developing this form of management and suspect it will be similar elsewhere. At this stage in the subject's development there is much scope for experiment but in the longer term there will have to be more formal training and appropriate examination and qualifications if nidotherapy is to become properly established.

Carers and helpers

There are many who take on a caring role for those with persistent mental illness who are in an admirable position to take on the role of nidotherapist. Such people may have few qualifications or have the task of caring foisted on them unprepared, as in the case of many close relatives, but when their responsibilities become established they can get to know the patient almost better than anybody else. They are thus in an excellent position to help the one who is being cared for by jointly planning environmental change.

CHAPTER 8

The place of nidotherapy in mental health services

It would be arrogant to assume that nidotherapy has any definite place in mental health services at this stage of its development but it clearly is more relevant to some areas than others. The diagnostic groups that might be considered are described in chapter 2; here we describe the services where it might be contemplated. It is already apparent from the earlier discussion about the indications for nidotherapy that acute services would have relatively little reason to consider nidotherapy in view of their focus on the management of presenting problems, but even here there may be a place for an environmental approach in acute manifestations of chronic conditions. However, most of the people who would naturally come to mind when thinking of nidotherapy are those who are in longer-term forms of care, many of which are subsumed under what is now called the recovery model.

The recovery and social models of mental illness

Models are used to fill in the gaps when data are missing and may be of value in establishing frameworks of intervention in psychiatric services, but despite their attraction they are not a substitute for data. The recovery model is a useful bridging concept that can be applied to help services that used to be clumsily described as 'the continuing care client' but in other parlance would be more simply described as 'chronic'. Across the globe we have neat sets of services for the ideal psychiatric patients who fit neatly into diagnostic groups, present to services in a predictable way and respond to treatment well. Where we fail is in providing similar slotted services for the complex people who make a nonsense of diagnosis and are confusingly described as having 'multiple comorbidity', who find psychiatric services unattractive or frankly odious, present there unwillingly after first going somewhere else, and make only a partial response to treatment, sometimes fighting it every step of the way. All these people can be incorporated into a loose recovery model, which thus covers a very heterogeneous group of people.

The recovery model

The essential components of the recovery model are really those of a positive philosophy that applies to everyone who comes for help to mental health services. Resnick *et al* (2004) identify four components that are intrinsic to this model: life satisfaction, hope and optimism, empowerment, and knowledge about mental illness and services. These components were derived from a large study, the Schizophrenia Patient Outcomes Research Team (PORT) and the patients who showed positive change in these areas were the ones who collectively were in the recovery group. Be that as it may, the notion that these patients have recovered in the conventional use of the term is not really accurate. It also assumes a position of conformity. Those people who did well took part in family education sessions, attended day hospital and legal services, and were generally cooperative. Many whom we consider for nidotherapy are the opposite of this: they are treatment resisting (see p. 61), oppose on principle, and are disdainful of any type of intervention that is aimed to 'make them better'. As one of our patients said to me in treatment early in the assessment for nidotherapy, 'I don't want to change my life, I just want you to give it back to me'.

The recovery model of care is assumed by most of the staff treating the individuals to have some of the central facets of what is commonly called the medical model of mental illness. This has been defined and redefined over the years but at its core carries the assumption that there is something wrong with the person that needs to be put right (i.e. the person is diagnosed with a mental disorder). Many in the recovery movement do not accept this premise, despite its acceptance by others (Mountain & Shah, 2008). The dissenters feel that hope, optimism and empowerment involves shaking off the shackles of some indefinable 'disorder', which tends to disempower and depress rather than encourage and promote health.

The social model

In the social model of mental illness (Tyrer & Steinberg, 2005) the assumptions are very different. This model regards all psychiatric diagnosis as unnecessary labelling which is stigmatising and disempowering. Independence and autonomy have been taken away by the diagnoser of the mental illness, and to add to the difficulties society also regards those with the disorder as either incompetent or vulnerable and handicaps them accordingly. This model, when taken to its extreme, regards illnesses such as schizophrenia to be a product of adverse social forces that prevent escape into sanity. As a comprehensive model of mental illness the social model clearly fails, but it is nearer to the core of nidotherapy than the recovery model. It agrees with nidotherapy in not wanting to change the person but to alter the immediate physical and social environment in a way that increases self-esteem, reduces any feelings of alienation and brings the person back from a mental health environment into a more normal and inclusive one.

Whichever model is chosen, the patients who might be considered for nidotherapy are likely to fall into one of four groups according to their service characteristics: chronic alienation, persistent resistance, therapeutic despair and what can only be described as the spinning, or rapidly revolving, door.

Chronic alienation

The people in this group do not feel they belong anywhere, not even among themselves. They cooperate to some extent with treatment but, for a variety of reasons, this does not seem to be effective or has so many negative aspects that it is rejected. As a consequence these people develop a cynical and detached attitude to treatment, expect it to fail and are less than active partners in any new therapeutic exercise. Because their attitudes and actions towards new approaches are so negative they tend to prove themselves right, so that every effort to improve things collapses like a pack of cards. Their alienation can be accentuated by the success of others with similar problems who do seem to make progress, which is doubly aggravating and makes the group even angrier.

Nidotherapy is not easy to introduce to this group, because even though it does not follow the lines of other therapies it tends to be damned by association. It is with this group that the ability to gain a trusting relationship is the best precursor to success, and this is one of the early goals in management.

Persistent resistance

People with persistent resistance are easy to identify. They are sometimes described as treatment-resistant but this is incorrect as they are primarily treatment resisting – they avoid treatment so actively that they cannot be described as having enough to demonstrate resistance to it. Nevertheless, the antipathy to intervention is so powerful that even when treatment is given the results tend to be poor, and if the condition is not one for which some form of coercion can be justified then the treatment cannot be given.

Nidotherapy has one big selling point in this group. It needs to be emphasised over and over again that it is not a treatment of the person but of the environment, so it is time for the patient to stop fighting and come to the negotiating table. This may be greeted with suspicion at first, because people in this group are very familiar with well-meaning clinicians who talk about treatment indirectly or in code as they realise that direct mention just provokes opposition. Again it is very important to develop a sufficient degree of trust to demonstrate that the nidotherapist has no hidden agenda and has no hidden therapeutic weapons waiting to be thrust onto the patient when no one is looking.

Therapeutic despair

This is probably the largest group to be considered for nidotherapy. Almost every form of mental disorder has the ability to become chronic and intractable, even when it seems a straightforward problem to treat at first. Although our recommendation is that it is only when a usually long-term course of treatment has failed that nidotherapy should be considered, the time when this point arrives is not always easy to determine. There is a natural determination for both therapist and patient to persist with treatment in one form or another until success is reached, but it is often clear when the tipping point has come and there is little chance of further success. 'Making the best of what you've got' could be a subtext for nidotherapy, but it is much more than that for this group. The tendency to persist with treatments, often demanding of resources for both patient and therapist, added to frequent adverse effects of the treatment in many cases, can become counterproductive. Nidotherapy offers a way out of the spiral of despair; it is not the patient who is not being abandoned but the treatment.

There are many ways of introducing nidotherapy at this point. The focus on the environment should not be interpreted as disinterest in treatment. Often existing treatment may be continued independently of nidotherapy and it can sometimes be argued that when the environmental changes have taken place the treatment may begin to work – an example of environment–treatment interaction that can only be positive when both elements are right. Nidotherapy also offers the opportunity of looking at the 'disorder' in a different light, more akin to the social model than a medical one. So in the case of a persistent depressive condition different questions can be asked: 'Do we have to consider this nasty problem as an illness?', 'Could it be a signal to you that there are many aspects of your life that are unsatisfactory and need attention?' These need not be spoken out loud, at least not at the beginning, but when nidotherapy is brought in as a way of looking at all the patient's difficulties in the round, as it were, there are many new perspectives that can be developed.

The spinning door

The spinning door rotates much more quickly than the revolving door, a much loved simile for those patients who frequently come back into psychiatric services, whether as an in-patient, out-patient or day patient, after apparently being set well on the road to full recovery. A 'revolving door' patient at least has a reasonable period when well, usually for many months, before relapse occurs for some reason. Those trapped in the spinning door are barely better before they become unwell again, and for everybody involved treatment is constantly chasing a new problem and never quite overcoming it. Some patients, particularly those with rapid cycling bipolar disorder, are natural spinners and for them it is reasonable to persist with both active and preventive treatments to both treat and prevent new episodes. But for many others it is impossible to say that the treatment is effective because relapse is so frequent.

It is more difficult to introduce nidotherapy to this group, as it is difficult to say that therapy has failed when it does seem to have short-term benefits. When environmental factors are clearly involved in the fluctuations there is an obvious reason for an environmental analysis, and again the possibility of negative environment–treatment interactions can be posited as reasons for relapse. Nidotherapy also gives the option of offering a broader view of a problem that tends to concentrate minds too much on the shorter-term benefits.

For all these groups and their attending services, nidotherapy has to be introduced carefully and often quite subtly. Established staff who have good therapeutic relationships with patients are not going to take kindly to a completely new approach, particularly one requiring their cooperation, unless it is handled sensitively and with full awareness of the special problems that might be posed from prior experience. In our own work the main concern expressed by other mental health professionals about nidotherapy is ignorance about the nature of the treatment with a worry that what might have been accomplished to date might be undone. Some of the major difficulties come when the normal service provision is recommended to be altered in a major way as a consequence of an agreed nidopathway. Thus, for example, a patient who had always been in supported accommodation because of risky behaviour was felt as a consequence of her nidotherapy assessment to be so keen on developing her own life without supervision (which she regarded as gross interference) that it was recommended that she should be given the opportunity to have an independent flat. As she was a person with a 'low flashpoint' to conflict and hated being in a crowded situation a flat was found that had a separate entrance from others in the building and which she could enter and leave without necessarily seeing any neighbours. This recommendation was implemented. A suitable flat was found and at the time of writing, 6 years later, she is still living there, not entirely without problems but with much less disturbance and a lot fewer admissions to hospital than when she was in allegedly safer and more expensive supported accommodation. This change in plan could not have been achieved without all members of the clinical team, the service manager, and indeed the senior manager covering the catchment area (in view of the patient's risk), approving of what started as a nidotherapy experiment but became a long-term element in the patient's care programme.

These changes in the service provision are only major for those patients with severe mental illness who use a great number of resources. The introduction of nidotherapy can be viewed as an unnecessary disturbance to a complex provision of care that should not be disturbed. However, where service providers should sit up and take notice is when they look at the cost savings achieved by nidotherapy in this group. It is not unreasonable to expect that if nidotherapy was included in rehabilitation services and did indeed enable people to find a better environmental fit, the amount of morbidity would reduce, as would the cost of care. Of course there will be exceptions where the nidotherapy assessment suggests a more expensive option than the one currently in place, but our research suggests the majority of placements would be cheaper.

The patients in this type of service would all be included in the recovery model as described above. Holloway (2008), in a perceptive analysis of the model, suggests that there are two different facets of the model, loosely characterised as the ordinary-language 'recovery-as-getting-better' and the contemporary conceptualisation of 'recovery as a journey of the heart', a deeply individual process that is linked with finding personal meaning even in the face of ongoing illness and disability'. Although these are separate elements and can change independently, nidotherapy addresses both. It does not directly attempt to get people better but by improving the fit between person and surroundings better harmony is introduced. The opportunities for personal growth and development within a favourable environment are so much greater than in an unfavourable one.

Development of nidotherapy in other mental care services

This book might be better entitled 'An Introduction to Nidotherapy', as our experience to date has only addressed a very small part of the population who might benefit from this approach. My clinical experience is reasonably broad but, as explained at the beginning of this book, nidotherapy developed out of despair at trying to provide something more positive to a population with not only severe mental illness but also 'triple diagnosis' (a combination of a psychosis, substance misuse and personality disorder). This represents only one part of the extreme end of the mental illness spectrum and it would be wrong to assume that nidotherapy has no place elsewhere.

Nidotherapy for carers and residential staff

Throughout this book I have emphasised the importance of developing a collaborative and trusting relationship with patients early in the course of nidotherapy and helping to ensure they play an active part in implementing suggested environmental changes. For many people with persistent mental health problems, including both children and adults with intellectual disability, the range of autistic spectrum disorders, Alzheimer's disease and other dementias, it is not usually possible to reach the desired degree of collaboration (this is not to say it should not be tried as it is very easy to assume wrongly that collaboration is lacking). The way of administering nidotherapy changes considerably under these circumstances.

Because a large proportion of the people in these groups need frequent care it is appropriate to concentrate on the carers, relatives, voluntary groups and others who provide most of the care and have, or at least should have, the greatest awareness of the person's needs. Here the aim is to practise a form of co-nidotherapy (p. 43) in which the carers are trained to become sensitive and effective nidotherapists. This can be a complex procedure, not least as there can be many carers involved with a single individual, and sometimes group training may be required.

Nidotherapy in other countries

Nidotherapy has been developed mainly in an overcrowded city (London) on an overpopulated island. This offers a restricted range of opportunities for environmental change and other places may well be able to exploit the principles of the treatment to greater advantage. In particular, the ability to achieve fundamentally different physical environments in one country (the best examples are probably Peru and Argentina) offers much greater scope. In low-income countries the abject squalor of the environments in which the poorest people live – graphically illustrated in Mumbai in the film *Slumdog Millionaire* (2008, by Danny Boyle and Looleen Tandan) – is an excellent illustration of how the absence of any encouragement in an environment can affect those who choose to stay rather than have at least the hope of attempting to escape. Ill-matching environments need not always be poverty-stricken. David Owen (2008) has coined the term 'hubris syndrome' to describe the problems of being in an environment in which almost every aspect of your physical, social and personal life is not only under your own control but can be manipulated almost any way you please. The outcome is that you can become cocooned in a universally positive reinforcing environment of your own making and then lose your critical faculties altogether, hence the hubris epithet. This adverse effect of too much nidotherapy can be true of despots and dictators but also of democratic leaders, and Owen suggests both George W. Bush and Tony Blair are world leaders who have manifested this condition.

One very positive aspect of nidotherapy for mental health services in low-income countries is that it is very cheap. No expensive equipment is necessary, no highly qualified specialists are required to administer it, and all that is needed is concentrated and focused human resources. There is also the potential for much greater flexibility in the opportunity for environmental changes when societies are more open. This is not true of all countries but where it is present there is much that nidotherapy can offer.

CHAPTER 9

The essentials of nidotherapy in four stages

There is pressure now for all treatments to be introduced in shortened form so that they can be planned and delivered within a specified time frame. This is not always appropriate – a collaborative treatment naturally sets its own timetable and external control in the form of rigid time control is not conducive to genuine collaboration.

Nevertheless, it is always useful to try and distil the essentials of a psychological treatment wherever possible as it can help to remove redundancies. This chapter therefore concentrates on the four core stages of nidotherapy that, if absolutely necessary and in less complex cases, may be concentrated into four sessions with a great deal of therapist homework to be carried out in between sessions. For more complex cases it will not be possible to complete a nidotherapy programme with this level of input but this period should be sufficient to at least create a nidotherapy strategy that enables others to continue the therapy afterwards. Longer-term therapy will be needed for fractious and temperamental patients who need to be cajoled and encouraged into treatment when it suits them, so many contacts may appear to be wasted at first. If encouraging and positive feedback is given whenever progress is made it may also build up a trusting alliance.

The duration of each of these stages can vary between 1 hour and many weeks, and contact with the patient can be supplemented by other sessions for training staff who are dealing with the patients concerned or with others such as relatives or friends. It is important to appreciate that if the sessions are to be reduced in number the amount of work to be carried out by the therapist will be increased. Most of this will be necessary between sessions but it can take many forms and it is better to think of the intervening periods between sessions as continuing treatment. Although the description of each component may suggest that only one session is needed, the reader should accommodate a much more flexible time frame when reading about each intervention. It is also assumed that the preliminary work described in chapter 2 has been carried out and that the patient is judged suitable for a nidotherapy intervention. Each of the sessions is accompanied by a checklist that may be useful as an *aide-memoire*.

Stage 1   Environmental analysis

Checklist:
1   Developing a trusting relationship with the patient as a person in his or her own preferred setting.
2   Determining which of the current problems are linked to the environment.
3   Analysis of environmental needs.
4   Assessment of changes necessary to achieve environmental needs.
5   Integration of needs.

1. Developing a trusting relationship with the patient as a person in his or her own preferred setting

Developing a good understanding of what the patient is really like is an essential component of nidotherapy and is perhaps one of the most difficult elements to learn. The best way to look at this is to think of the person being treated as an actor in many different plays. In each role he or she, often unwittingly, carries out predictable responses. Often these are not fundamental core components of that person's behaviour, but the setting over the years in which they have been developed makes behaviour and attitudes stereotyped and not really a reflection of the real person. The job of the nidotherapist is to 'get inside the skin' of the person being treated, not in an analytical or devious way but as an open and direct effort to understand how the person really thinks and feels. This is a necessary universal part of nidotherapy discussed in previous chapters. Being a good listener is an important, almost essential, part of this process. Almost certainly in the past there will have been occasions when therapists have assumed they know what a particular patient is thinking with regard to their environment and made decisions in the light of this. It is sad to summarise many of these as wrong-headed or inappropriate, mainly because they assume a belief or set of wishes that is transplanted to their patient from their own ways of thinking. This may sometimes be right, but for most of the people being considered for nidotherapy it is probably wrong and as the choice may not lead to the improvement expected.

So when I, as an irritable consultant under time pressure, interrupt a patient on the grounds that I have worked out everything the patient wants and needs, and nothing more that is useful can be gained by continuing the conversation, I need to check myself and show a bit more humility, and then listen a bit more carefully.

Making assumptions as to what is most needed may have to be considered when the environmental way forward is unclear, but only when the views of all relevant parties, and most especially the patient, have been heard.

2. Determining which of the current problems are linked to the environment

Once there is a reasonable degree of trust in the early stage of nidotherapy it should be possible to find out which of the problems demonstrated or expressed are linked to the environment and which ones are independent. This is an essential distinction and additional corroborative evidence from other health workers or from written records may be of use here. The identification of these may not always help in determining the long-term nidotherapy plan but they do indicate the areas of concern that will need to be explored. If this goes well it may also be possible to establish the central unchanging aspects of the problems that need environmental change in order to overcome them, and this can be the beginning of the nidopathway.

3. Analysis of environmental needs

In this first stage it should be possible to identify some environmental needs and the therapist may then have some glimmerings as to which of these, or of other secondary ones, may be core needs worthy of the planned nidopathway. Let us take a common example to see how one need can illustrate a core issue (Case study 9.1).

Case study 9.1

A patient with schizophrenia and suicidal ideas (and previous attempts) was placed in a high-support hostel. He seemed settled at first but after a few weeks became more and more difficult in his engagement with the staff at the hostel and was irritable and aggressive when they did see him. The nidotherapist asked to inter-vene decided to see him first at the hostel and in the course of the initial session they had a frank discussion. The patient explained that the cause of his irritation was the lack of warning given by the hostel staff when they came to see him in his room, and their consequent impatience if he was not ready immediately. This was then illustrated by a long set of other complaints over the lack of respect for his privacy and autonomy, of which this was only one example. 'I'm a grown man but they treat me like a 5-year-old,' he said, 'and I know they're making sure I'm not suicidal but their constant checking on me is making me more suicidal, so it's obviously not working.' 'More autonomy' was therefore identified as a general core environmental need in this first session.

If a set of needs is presented in this first stage they will obviously be looked at individually but should also be examined for common features that might be solved by a single environmental change. It is always better to get beyond the particular to the general at this stage of assessment. At the end of this assessment the nidotherapist will have, either literally or just in mind, an idea of those issues that are likely to be persistent and permanent, those that are clearly temporary, and another group of which it is impossible to be certain.

4. Assessment of changes necessary to achieve environmental needs

Once needs have been identified, no matter how vaguely, it is possible to explore the options for environmental change, even including those that might be quite impracticable. It quickly becomes clear that it is not worth making major changes in the environment to help to solve a problem that is only present for a short time. Nevertheless, a transient problem, if recurrent, may lead to constant handicap and be worthy of nidotherapy. Thus, an ambitious person wishing to better him- or herself may persistently fail at interviews because of increased anxiety and consequent poor performance. A standard method of dealing with this problem would be to treat what is commonly called 'social anxiety' using a variety of methods. If initial enquiry shows considerable doubt in the person's mind about promotion and its implications this may become an indication for nidotherapy where a less stressful environment is decided on as the main goal.

The consideration of alternatives also needs to be explored with the patient openly and freely, not least because a list of environmental complaints can easily become a litany that is self-defeating if it is not leavened by some constructive options. In doing this it is helpful to look at the problem from a different angle in an imaginative way, possibly one that has not been considered before. Thus a woman who persistently complained that she did not have the resources to do what she always wanted, to paint in oils, was introduced to a service linked to an art gallery project where she was not only allowed, but also encouraged and helped directly with judicious supervision to develop her talents. Even those options chosen by the patient that are clearly not feasible at least should merit some discussion and a mutual agreement should be reached for them to be dropped and, where possible, to be resurrected at a later date.

The discussion can also take into account the current treatment plan and how it would fit in with the proposed environmental changes, which will also help to establish that the patient is suitable for nidotherapy at this stage of their problem. Some problems may appear to be long lasting and apparently permanent but are still being addressed by different treatments in the hope that benefits will ensue. In these situations it is wise not to introduce nidotherapy. Again the reason is not difficult to elucidate. The decision to take on someone for nidotherapy is an admission that both existing and future treatments are unlikely to have a fundamental impact on the progress of the condition. Of course, this does not mean that all treatments should be abandoned, but certainly for the period of nidotherapy the expectation would be that any new treatment will either have limited benefit or take a long time before it is shown to be of value. It is important not to choose nidotherapy as an easy option if all possible treatments have not been considered carefully.

5. Integration of needs

By the end of this stage there should be a clear indication of the nature and extent of the environmental problems that are concerning the patient, what changes are likely to be long-lasting, which changes are core, and what interventions are likely to be feasible and successful. The last two may only be decided in a rough and provisional form, and both therapist and patient may wish to work on them in more detail before the start of the next session.

Exercise 9.1

A patient who has many different problems and is said to have 'complex co-morbidities' is referred for nidotherapy. He has schizophrenic symptoms that are largely related to taking cannabis resin, considerable social anxiety (which initially led him to take cannabis) and occasionally attacks of panic. He has no close relationships apart from that with his family.

Describe how you would determine whether nidotherapy is indicated and the areas of likely focus for nidotherapy if it is offered.

Stage 2   Making the nidopathway

Checklist:
1   Provisional pathway
2   Environmental testing and planned environmental change
3   Person feedback
4   Formulation of final pathway and what resources are available

1. Provisional pathway

In the second stage, the first interventional component of nidotherapy begins. This is the analysis of the environment in all its forms and how it might be altered to benefit the patient. This sounds a great deal easier in theory than it actually is in practice, largely because environmental needs are not always shining forth like beacons waiting to be tackled. They are often hidden under other problems and have to be exposed in this session of treatment.

2. Environmental testing and planned environmental change

Environmental testing has to be linked to planned changes in the environment in this phase. If there is doubt about whether a change is likely to prove beneficial it may be necessary to test out at least one of its components. Thus a man who cannot decide whether he is capable of sharing supported accommodation – something he is attracted to as he has always been lonely living alone in the past – could be placed for an experimental period in a shared setting, supervised closely during this time, and a decision made at the end of the test period.

3. Person feedback

Although person feedback is a desirable element at all stages of nidotherapy, it is particularly important at this stage. A lot of different changes may be possible but many will have to be rejected if they cannot be implemented easily or the patient is opposed to them. Sometimes this opposition may be inappropriate or only lightly held, in which case it is important to explore how much leeway may be present in adjusting or altering these views collaboratively so that they are not perceived as imposed conditions.

These views can often be identified by apparent incongruities. Thus we saw a patient recently who said she had never been liked by anybody. Later in the interview she referred to a short time in her life when she was working, possibly in a fairly menial job but was respected for her contribution and treated in a completely different way from how she had been before and after this time. So the question beginning with 'Is it really true that you have never …' referring to a persistent catalogue of negative events and responses may elicit the one positive answer that allows an opening to be made in advance of setting the nidotherapy targets.

4. Formulation of final pathway and what resources are available

Once a way forward is found, the help of many others is likely to be needed before it can be implemented. The nidotherapist should therefore look to possible allies the patient might be able to draw on in tackling the problems. Some of these may be obvious, such as family and friends, but others may be professionals, teachers or neighbours who might not normally be thought of in these terms. Other resources include financial ones such as statutory benefits, and others may be forms of emotional support that could be of immense potential value. In thinking of environmental needs it is easy just to take a short-term perspective. Many people may feel they can 'help out' but not provide any form of long-term input. If one of the environmental needs is a social one it is important to be absolutely certain that it is reasonably robust before introducing it into any subsequent programme.

Exercise 9.2

A young woman living in a poor housing estate suffers from 'chronic depression and irritability' and blames all her troubles on her environment, hence her referral

Exercise 9.2 *Continued*

for nidotherapy. The first stage of assessment seems to be straightforward. She needs to be in a better area and describes what it would be like to wake up in a flat with eye-catching furniture, matching walls and ceilings, and all utilities working well; she cannot understand why all her efforts to achieve this goal fail persistently. She shows an element of apparent paranoia in pointing to other people in a similar situation who have succeeded in getting much better accommodation and feels she is being discriminated against. In exploring the reasons why she is not able to achieve this aim, two possible openings are identified. The first is that she is estranged from her family after having violent arguments with them before leaving home. From indirect comments it appears that her family are still positive about her and would like to establish contact again, and they also may have the resources to support her in getting better accommodation. Second, one of the reasons why she has not been able to move to a more appropriate flat is persistent accumulation of arrears because of her poor budgeting.

It is concluded that more satisfactory accommodation satisfying many of her needs may be within reach and is not an unrealistic want.

Describe how you would go about achieving better accommodation for the patient, what obstacles you are likely to experience, and how you would overcome them.

Stage 3   Initiating change

Checklist:
1   Starting on the right foot
2   Reinforcing progress
3   Reviewing the timetable
4   Adjusting targets and responsibilities
5   Resetting timetables

1. Starting on the right foot

The first two stages of this exercise establish the framework for environmental change. This may surprise some people as it might be thought wise to get the modifications to the environment established long before the halfway stage. Effecting change is a stage of nidotherapy that many feel should come early on after the treatment is explained. This would be a mistake because the two earlier sessions are essential in developing the level of consensus that allows agreement of targets to be reached at this stage. After the first two sessions of treatment we have a much clearer idea of what environmental changes are necessary and these may be very different from those that were identified at the beginning. Almost always this will represent a consensus of views in which those of both therapist and patient have changed markedly from their original ideas. By the time we get to session four the general notion of what should be done has been developed; what is needed now is to put clear substance on these ideas and make them into practical goals.

A wide range of specific suggestions for environmental change will be discussed here and although it is not considered necessary to write down much of the details of discussions in previous sessions, it is probably wise to summarise the targets in writing at the end of this stage so that they are unambiguous. Even at this stage it may not be possible to be as firm as one would like to be about exactly what these targets are. They can be expressed in relatively vague language (e.g. 'to live somewhere else') in which the exact form of the environmental change has yet to be clearly specified.

It is also useful at this stage to clarify those environmental wishes (wants) that cannot be attained during nidotherapy. This may be because they are considered inappropriate or they are impracticable within a reasonable timescale, or they are appropriate but cannot possibly be attained for a variety of other reasons. Such clarification is helpful to make sure the patient does not feel that his or her views have been ignored or bypassed in the nidotherapy programme.

2. Reinforcing progress

Once the targets have been agreed upon – and it is probably wise not to have more than three or four identified unless they are clearly linked – the pathways to achieving them need to be formulated. This may lead to definitive or sketchy pathways, but it cannot be forgotten or dismissed. At the risk of bombarding readers with unnecessary neologisms, the term 'nidopathway' is described for this process in Tyrer & Bajaj (2005), as although there may be many other pathways towards the achievement of targets in nidotherapy, the nidopathway is specific to the individual target. Thus, for example, one of the common conclusions of the first part of this session is a set of three targets: a change of accommodation; more autonomy to be allowed in the person's life; and the selection of new and more interesting spare-time activities. The nidopathway for the first target is largely an administrative negotiated one that will involve the therapist in doing a great deal of work as well as getting guidance from the patient. A second nidopathway will involve more responsibility being taken by the patient and may well include a set of environmental experiments whereby greater autonomy is given to make sure that the risks of granting these can be properly assessed. A third nidopathway involves even more decision-making by the patient. One of the big problems people with severe mental illness experience is having too much spare time and prolonged periods of boredom. And sadly this is often dealt with in practice by looking for stimulation in the form of illicit drugs rather than other, more appropriate and healthy activities. This nidopathway may well be a tortuous one and may involve many different attempts to get satisfaction before a target is finally achieved. So for this person we will have three nidopathways – focusing on accommodation, autonomy and spare time – that are virtually independent and have to be monitored separately. One of these may be considered much more important than all others and at various times the others may be suspended so as to allow more attention to be given to the main one, but throughout this discussion there needs to be a good level of consensus, with both parties agreeing on changes and adjustments.

The role of arbitrage may also be important in this session. This is formulated as one of the key principles of nidotherapy (Tyrer *et al*, 2003*a*) and involves choosing an arbiter who enjoys the full confidence of both therapist and patient and whose judgement will be accepted by both parties. If nidotherapy proceeds well it may not be necessary to have an arbiter but it is likely that at some point during the negotiations between therapist and patient there will be considerable difficulties in getting agreement. For this reason it is useful to have an arbiter identified at this stage if one is available. Of course for those who have very little support in their lives it may be impossible to get a suitable arbiter, but it is surprising how often one can be chosen in advance when this possibility is seriously looked at.

3. Reviewing the timetable

This is a useful but not absolutely essential component of phase three. To some extent the timetable has already been brought into the discussion in deciding on the targets for nidotherapy, because if the achievement of a target is likely to take many years it is unlikely to appear in the list that is being developed. For many of the targets it is almost impossible to decide on a timetable, whereas for some it becomes essential. Thus, for example, if it is decided to think of new accommodation for someone who has large rent arrears in their present accommodation and cannot move until these have been settled, then the target either has to be abandoned or a clear pathway developed for paying off the arrears.

4. Adjusting targets and responsibilities

In this part of the programme it is often clear that there are many tasks that need to be carried out and only some of these require specialised skills. One of the easy options, and one that is unfortunately pursued by many in ordinary practice, is to say that the patient should carry out these tasks themselves as he or she is going to get the major benefits from their completion. The assumption is then made that the person concerned has the ability and wherewithal to carry out the tasks without much in the way of external assistance. For those with severe mental illness this is often a crass assumption. Incompetence breeds incompetence and in the absence of reward reinforcement is rare. The other option of the nidotherapist taking on all these tasks is seldom wise. One of the problems that can develop is the fostering of excessive dependence so that when the time comes for treatment to end disengagement becomes very difficult. It is also necessary to try and develop a framework whereby any gains made during nidotherapy can be sustained afterwards when a formal intervention has ceased.

For this reason it is wise to get as many helpers as possible on board the nidotherapy ship, so that it can complete all its tasks before it docks. These can include relatives, other staff in clinical teams and units, volunteers, friends and acquaintances. One of the unfortunate consequences of long-term mental health difficulties is isolation and disengagement from others. Gentle exploration often reveals that such disengagement is not total and some re-establishing of links is often possible.

In carrying out these tasks it is also important to keep the patient aware and in at least some control of the developing situation. One of the major problems in the past, perhaps most obvious in the Victorian age of paternalism, is that other well-meaning people decide what environmental changes are necessary for a specific individual without any form of proper consultation. Unless the patient is kept in touch with what is being planned and gives at least tacit approval to the plans, they are likely to go awry.

In setting these tasks there is a need for overall coordination and integration. Clearly some of the tasks will fail for reasons that have nothing to do with the efforts of the people concerned, but others will fail because promises are not kept and those who are faint hearted will not persist in completing the tasks. What is sometimes needed to break the impasse in progress is a small element of extra help from the nidotherapist. This can be looked on as unnecessary (as most of the tasks concerned can be done without help) but such actions increase the feelings of partnership with the patient and in this session one could be included. A good example is provided below (Case study 9.2).

This kind of help can become a springboard to solve other areas of isolation – contact with the person's family, establishing further voluntary work, taking part in communal support activities – but the first often needs a special push from someone other than the patient. Sometimes the help can be given with the patient looking on, so that the opportunity of mimicry or modelling is shown, when the nidotherapy will overlap with behaviour therapy.

Of course, if only one session is going to be available for this phase of nidotherapy, other people may be needed to act as facilitators to achieve the same ends. This type of adjustment in a planned nidopathway can often be

---

Case study 9.2

Graham had personality features of impulsiveness and anger and was repeatedly banned from the services in his area because he was always perceived as threatening and potentially dangerous. In discussion with his nidotherapist it became clear that his life was very impoverished by all these exclusions but he was quite incapable of avoiding losing his temper when the slightest bit aggravated. With the help of his nidotherapist he was eventually allowed to work on an allotment shared by other patients in the service and a policy was worked out by which his aggressive feelings, when aroused, were converted into digging the plot or other tasks that expressed his anger in a more appropriate way.

one of the anticipatory actions to be implemented if a target is not achieved: 'If you are not able to do this as we hope you can, we will then add some extra help so that you will be able to get it done', and then the extra help is spelled out.

5. Resetting timetables

In a limited number of sessions there will be insufficient time to set a new timetable for new targets in nidotherapy. The best that can be done at this stage is to discuss the options available if the initial plan is less than successful. Alternatively, only a vague timetable is put forward at this point in therapy and the opportunity of firming this up at a later date is given.

Exercise 9.3

Malcolm is a farmer who has developed chronic depression but has not responded to antidepressants and is scornful of psychological therapies. Environmental analysis suggests that he has become demoralised by the same system of dairy and arable farming that he has been involved with ever since leaving school and which is yielding fewer and fewer returns. It is suggested that he needs a new challenge in his work and after looking at the options he is attracted to the challenge of looking after South American llamas and is very impressed by the high price of llama wool. He buys four llamas after some encouragement from the nidotherapist.

Describe how you would monitor the nidopathway and Malcolm's depression in a way that could satisfy the hypothesis that his work style was the main factor reinforcing his depression.

Stage 4   Long-term planning

Checklist:
1   Confirming a final nidopathway
2   Planning longer-term environmental change
3   Getting agreement from all parties
4   Anticipating problems
5   Setting responsibilities for the future

This stage will be the easiest of the four if the remainder have gone smoothly. If only four sessions have been set aside for the nidotherapy. the last stage will be used to review the progress made and to plan a much longer but more leisured pathway to the goals of treatment. The philosophy of the approach should be well understood by the patient now and help from others – such as potential co-nidotherapists (p. 43) – can be discussed in monitoring further progress. Anticipation of problems can never be comprehensive but it is useful to discuss them and to work towards resolving them in general terms without necessarily providing prescriptive solutions.

In Case study 9.3 a 10-year-long nidopathway is described to illustrate the essentials of all four stages of nidotherapy.

Case study 9.3 The case of the restless tenant (to illustrate nidotherapy in four stages)

Henry was a 37-year-old man who had been homeless for several periods in the past and had long been suspicious of the intentions of others. Through the efforts of the special homelessness team who originally treated him in central London he was eventually given a flat. Despite being pleased at first, he was unhappy with several aspects of the environment. He complained repeatedly to the council and was moved to another flat, and shortly afterwards, to yet another. On the surface this all appeared to be due to noise. Henry was very sensitive to noise (and had very good hearing) but the problems he felt about noise were not in his view an accident of nature. He was convinced that the city council were housing him in unsatisfactory noisy accommodation as a deliberate policy. He eventually came round to believing that the senior housing officers in the council were specifically targeting him and making sure that he always had the least appropriate property for his needs. He became very frustrated by the way the housing department dealt with his problems and almost invariably finished up shouting at them for their incompetence and inadequacy. As Henry had a very loud voice this type of encounter often led to trouble, and frequently the police were called when he became angry about these issues in the housing department itself. He had been admitted to hospital on two occasions and diagnosed as having a persistent delusional disorder (i.e. a diagnosis within the schizophrenia group of diagnoses which is made when people have single persistent delusions but no other features indicative of schizophrenia). He received an antipsychotic drug in low dosage, as much for its sedative value as for any antipsychotic effects, but this had very little impact and it was soon withdrawn. It was clear at the end of three interviews with Henry that he was in a position to qualify for the receipt of nidotherapy (stage 1). He had also developed a degree of trust in the new assessment as no presuppositions about what was necessary had been made.

At the environmental analysis that accompanies the second phase it became clear that Henry was primarily preoccupied by noise. As his flat was in central London, and as he was dependent on a property base available for vulnerable people who did not have the resources to pay, it was clear that the level of noise that he wished for was unlikely to be attained. In the first instance he was moved from a very noisy and unsatisfactory flat that needed renovating to another one not far away that at first seemed to be satisfactory. This also had a small garden and Henry was assisted by members of the nidotherapy team in helping to make this more attractive and a personally satisfying place to be in. However, before long he was increasingly concerned about noises in the flat above and particularly complained about what appeared to be the movement of heavy furniture in the early hours of the morning.

At this point an important decision was made. The nidotherapist persuaded Henry that it was probably inappropriate for him to negotiate with the housing department about the problem as he would almost certainly lose his temper with them, 'have a rant' and be forcibly removed from the premises. It was agreed that the clinical team (an assertive outreach team) would be allowed to act as arbiter in negotiating with the housing department. This was an important breakthrough and

---

Case study 9.3 *(contd)*

has been maintained ever since (over a period of 6 years to date). In investigating the problem of heavy furniture being moved in the night, it transpired that Henry was entirely correct. The flat upstairs was being used as business premises and the activities often involved working at unsocial hours. Close enquiry revealed that a heavy photocopier was often moved in the early hours of the morning in order to make space for other activities and a complaint about this was duly made. Unfortunately little progress was made in reducing the nocturnal activities of the business concerned but Henry felt vindicated because his concerns were backed up by his nidotherapist and the clinical team and he no longer felt isolated and negotiating on his own.

At the end of the equivalent of stage 2 of the nidotherapy programme (seven sessions in the case of Henry) we had identified which of his environmental needs were important, which were inappropriate (i.e. a noiseless environment), and how it might be possible to achieve some of his ends by negotiating on his behalf. The resources of the clinical team were also brought into play in this enterprise.

The plan was therefore developed by which continued contact was maintained with a specific aim of helping adjustment in Henry's current flat and no longer addressing what were formally his mental health needs (i.e. paranoid symptoms and aggression towards the housing department). This was a much more harmonious relationship than his previous ones with mental health services, which had frequently ended up with Henry dismissing well-intentioned people who had been delegated to help him because they didn't understand what his problems were and magnified them by colluding with the people who were causing them. This made the sessions very different from how they were originally. Instead of visiting Henry and receiving a long, virtually uninterrupted, rant about all the things that were going wrong, we had a friendly discussion about progress that needed to be made, or was already being made, exploring aspects such as noise reduction and housing negotiations, and this was achieved with a measure of trust and understanding that had never been formerly attained. In none of these meetings was it necessary to ask direct questions about Henry's mental state or aspects of treatment because this was clearly irrelevant to the main task at hand. From time to time there were difficulties because of the occasionally angry exchange that Henry had with members of the housing department but these were kept to a minimum and detailed discussion with the department allowed much greater understanding on their part as to the real nature of Henry's problems. By the end of this period it was clear that specific nidotherapy input was coming to an end because Henry was able to do more positively with colleagues in the housing department and a much greater level of understanding had been achieved with them.

This period covers stages 3 and 4 in the earlier descriptions. The tasks that were necessary to explore Henry's environment became clear and focused and were agreed by everybody concerned in the assessments. This involved the nidotherapist with many more tasks than would be expected in the average mental health consultation. Indeed, by the end of this session it would have been impossible for almost all observers to know that Henry's problems were primarily those of mental ill health because this subject was never mentioned.

Over the past 4 years Henry has continued to make good progress. He has moved once more but this was a planned and considered move and he has a fulfilling

Case study 9.3 *(contd)*

range of activities that have created contentment. From time to time he still has worries about some of his neighbours but most of these are dealt with easily through his contact (not frequent) with the clinical team. He only sees his nido-therapist occasionally for what could be regarded as booster sessions but these really constitute updates on aspects of his home adjustment. At the end of treatment we have someone whose mental state is basically unchanged but who feels tuned in to those around him and in particular that he has a network of people who can help him whenever things go wrong. This network understands him and has the same perspective on his problem as he does, which reassures him greatly and adds to his level of trust.

What has happened over the course of the nidotherapy programme is that Henry has achieved what is now commonly called 'social inclusion' – he is accepted in his microcosm of society and accepts others to a much greater extent than he ever did before. He has not changed – but he has become well.

CHAPTER 10

Questions and answers

In this chapter we hope to satisfy the puzzlement of many who come to nidotherapy either for the first time or after trying the approach in practice. There are some who do not share our enthusiasm and just think of nidotherapy as old wine in new bottles, or just plain common sense, unnecessarily bottled and packaged when it is more comfortable out in the open. Time after time we come back to the core aim of nidotherapy – to change the environment to make the best possible fit for the patient and not to attempt to change the person directly – and we do not know of any other strategies or treatments that have the same primary aim. But we appreciate there are bound to be many questions about this form of management. Some have been asked repeatedly in the academic settings where nidotherapy has been described but there must be many more. The answers that are given below may satisfy some of the concerns, and even if they do not always do so, they should in particular show that the treatment adds something beyond the procedures of normal practice.

Is nidotherapy a psychological treatment?

Yes. Although it is clearly specified as an intervention that changes the environment, it does this in collaboration with the patient. This collaboration is very rarely a straightforward exercise such as meeting the bank manager and arranging a loan for a specific purpose, as it does not just satisfy a specific, exact environmental need but involves a full analysis of all aspects of the environment and careful judgement of the options afterwards. The processes involved require psychological skills that overlap with other psychotherapies but which are used in a different way. Sometimes nidotherapy has to be given indirectly without much direct contract with the patient, but more often it involves the development of a relationship and rapport with someone who is not exactly sure of their environmental wishes and whose needs require refining and developing in the context of a trusting relationship. This process requires skills that constitute psychological therapy.

Is there any difference between nidotherapy and good clinical care using a comprehensive treatment approach?

Yes, there is. Comprehensive treatment plans, such as the full implementation of the care management approach in the UK, include an assessment of environmental and well as personal needs, and this can overlap with nidotherapy. The difference between these approaches and nidotherapy is that in nidotherapy the environmental analysis and subsequent intervention are planned and systematic. It focuses solely on the environment in all its forms and assumes, sometimes incorrectly and pessimistically, that the person being treated is not going to change with regard to the essentials of their mental state. By not being diverted into changing people's symptoms, nidotherapy gets a full run at the environment in a way that is rarely allowed in other forms of care. Instead of being satisfied by a rough approximation to environmental wishes and a combination of acceptance of the patient's situation with a desire to change in terms of attitudes and symptom relief, nidotherapy unashamedly goes for environmental change only, and by so doing makes advances that would be regarded as unattainable using other approaches. We used the example of Janet Frame in the Foreword of this book, but we can also point to the almost complete recovery of patients with apparently chronic and intractable illness by getting the right environmental fit. Many of these cases are discussed (with minor changes to avoid identification) elsewhere in this book but what should also be clear is that the fundamental nature of the mental illness has not altered with any of these people.

Can nidotherapy be given to a completely uncooperative patient?

Yes. Although it is desirable for good engagement to be in place for nidotherapy to be implemented, it can be done by proxy or by other indirect means. The environmental analysis can be done using a combination of observation, written records (preferably over a long timescale), and details of interactions with a wide variety of people, and changes made in the environment as a consequence of this analysis. This suggested nidopathway can then be monitored as for standard nidotherapy with willing patients.

Is it ethical to give nidotherapy to people without informing them about it?

This is a difficult question, but since in one way or another everybody takes notice of the environment in their daily life, it is reasonable to proceed on the basis that it is sometimes ethical to make an environmental change without full discussion beforehand, provided that it is explained fully at a later date. For those who do not have capacity to understand (e.g. those with severe intellectual disability, dementia, delirium; see e.g. Meagher *et al*, 1996), others will have to take on the role of consent and full discussion is necessary in these instances. Planned rather than forced environmental change is always preferable.

For what problems is nidotherapy contraindicated?

Nidotherapy should not be attempted when there is a temporary disruption in psychological functioning that may distort decision-making. To take an obvious example, a successful businessman who becomes severely depressed may regard himself as useless and a fraud, and if going through an environmental analysis may conclude that he should sell his business and live in modest squalor as this is the most that he deserves. This plan could be generated collaboratively and smoothly with a nidotherapist but would almost certainly be regretted afterwards when the depression was reversed. For this reason, when dealing with psychological problems of recent onset or with previous evidence of resolution, nidotherapy should be postponed until it is clear that other therapies have run their course and have no further increments of effectiveness.

Are 'psychopaths' appropriate for nidotherapy?

The term 'psychopath' is an unfortunate one because it covers a great deal of pathology that is not homogeneous and covers aspects of antisocial personality disorder, personal opportunism, self-importance and criminal behaviour. However, the term now is commonly used for those who have a high score on the Psychopathy Checklist (PCL) (Hare, 1991), a 20-item checklist that identifies glib, plausible, unfeeling and exploitative people who may appear to cooperate well in treatment but do so only to achieve their own ends, ones that are quite separate from those of the therapy. There is some evidence that this is particularly true with psychological treatments (Shine & Hobson, 2000) and so the true collaborative relationship necessary for nidotherapy could be subverted.

In practice it is important for the nidotherapist to liaise with others who know the patient, both to be appraised of developments that may not otherwise be disclosed and to get feedback about possible environmental plans that may seem feasible but are inappropriate for other reasons; put more simply, the therapist must avoid being conned. At the same time, it becomes very difficult for those who have antisocial and psychopathic personality features to convince others that they are acting genuinely, if there is persistent scepticism about their motives whenever they appear to be doing the right thing.

Can drug and psychological treatments be combined with nidotherapy?

Yes, but usually as maintenance rather than new therapies. Nidotherapy is unable to be practised if there are constant fluctuations in the mental status of the person, as these almost invariably interfere with the process of treatment. Symptomatic change is not in itself a problem, but attitudes, behaviour and judgements often change also and this does interfere with nidotherapy as environmental plans and agreements often fluctuate in tandem with them. Nevertheless, there are many ways in which other treatments can interact positively with nidotherapy. Patients with schizophrenia who make a good response to antipsychotic drug treatment but keep on defaulting on maintenance treatment may be referred for nidotherapy when this pattern of consequences persists.

If interference in environmental adjustment is recognised as related to stopping drug treatment, a new reason for continuing drug therapy can be identified that is often seen as more appropriate than the standard instruction 'You have to continue this medication, otherwise you will relapse and have to come back into hospital'. Nidotherapy approaches adherence to drug treatment not from the direct treatment angle but from the environmental one. In discussing environmental needs the question of drug treatment can arise in a more positive way. Thus a patient with marked paranoid symptoms who feels threatened by dozens of dangers whenever he steps outside his flat can identify taking an antipsychotic drug as an environmental aid – 'When I take the tablet the world doesn't seem as hostile'.

Similarly, patients who are crippled by persistent anxiety and cannot focus on psychological forms of treatment because they get distracted and distressed so readily, once involved with nidotherapy and feeling more at home in a preferred setting, can be engaged in psychological treatments such as cognitive–behavioural therapy. In crossing the boundary between nidotherapy and other treatments it is imperative to make the distinction between the treatment of the environment and the treatment of the patient clear to both nidotherapist and patient. If the two become blurred this creates unnecessary confusion.

Can nidotherapy be followed by new forms of treatment?

Yes. This is an important question to answer because at first sight it may appear that nidotherapy is the treatment at the end of the road and subsequently there is nothing more that can be done. It would be a mistake to think this because nidotherapy may unblock many of the obstacles that have prevented the patient from responding to other forms of treatment. The situation is rather like a horse in a steeplechase. One of the fences may prove too difficult to negotiate so the horse pulls up. However, if niodtherapy enables the horse to go round the obstacle and join the course again it can then negotiate the other fences. Case study 10.1 illustrates this change.

Is nidotherapy better for problems that have a psychological cause?

No. Nidotherapy is completely disinterested in the specific cause of a mental problem, although it does like to know if the problem is likely to resolve spontaneously or show progressive deterioration. Because of this it

> **Case study 10.1**
>
> A 35-year-old man had a diagnosis of schizophrenia and perpetually fought against this label because he did not consider he had the condition. He therefore repeatedly failed to maintain treatment as an out-patient and came back into hospital within 3 months of being discharged. When seen for nidotherapy the question of his medication was not directly addressed but in the course of assessment he commented that he felt safe only at home and that almost everyone outside his flat seemed to be against him. In working out what might enable him to feel more comfortable in his surroundings, one of the factors identified was the short period when he was out of hospital before he began to relapse. In analysing this together with the therapist, the patient had a glimmering of recognition that the taking of medication was one of the reasons why he felt more at home shortly after he was discharged from hospital. This was developed further in his nidotherapy programme until the taking of medication was regarded as part of the nidotherapy management. Put another way, the taking of medication was recognised to be an environmentally desirable change and therefore qualifies as an appropriate intervention. Obviously it happened to be a therapeutic intervention as well, but because it was approached from the environmental angle much of the adversarial aspect of taking medication was avoided.

can often be useful when treating a person with a condition in which there is doubt about the cause and thereby the treatment. For example, chronic fatigue syndrome is a subject that arouses a great deal of emotion, as some people feel it is a neurological syndrome with a clear biological cause, whereas others feel it can be more appropriately classified as a psychological disorder. To recommend psychological treatment for this disorder is seen as tantamount to supporting the second argument and the personal consequences of this are outlined graphically by Wessely and his colleagues (1998) in their account of the problem. Nidotherapy does not take sides on the cause of a particular problem, it merely says 'You are where you are, we do not know exactly how you got here, but let us see if we can make things better for you by changing your environment'. No questions are asked about cause, no answers are needed and no feathers are ruffled.

How do you deal with a set of environmental requirements that are clearly inappropriate or unattainable?

Unrealistic aims are frequent at the beginning of nidotherapy. At first many are awash in amazement amidst the luxury of being actually asked unconditionally what changes they want in their environment. This is such a difference from the standard barked order to do something you know not what or why, and so it is not surprising that the invitation for the patient to make their own suggestions goes a little to the head, and odd ideas are born. These need to be explored gently but not dismissed out of hand, and by the time the discussion is finished the person will have been convinced that there are more practical alternatives that should be explored first.

The advantage of an independent arbiter is also valuable here. If it is impossible to get agreement between nidotherapist and patient, it is a great relief to be able to turn to a person who is respected by both sides and whose decision is accepted as final.

Can you practise nidotherapy without previous experience in mental health?

Yes, but it would be unwise to do this completely unsupervised. In the early stages of nidotherapy the decision whether to persist with treatment of a long-standing condition or to abandon the effort as fruitless and turn to nidotherapy is a difficult one to make, and really cannot be done without considerable knowledge of the course and different forms of management of mental illness. But with supervision and guidance these decisions can be made by others and the other skills necessary for a nidotherapist outlined in chapter 7 may be present without a good background in mental health. For less serious disorders there is no reason why self-nidotherapy should not be tried. This merely involves people making their own environmental analyses dispassionately, sometimes with the help of loved ones, friends or relatives, and then implementing the decisions accordingly. What are commonly called 'lifestyle changes' could be included here.

How do you know when nidotherapy has failed?

Nidotherapy is a collaborative enterprise. Both patient and therapist are monitoring its progress and when both recognise that nothing of value is happening the therapy could be regarded as having failed. However, there is a difference between outright failure and a temporary halt. Nidotherapy may fail because an expected environmental change fails to materialise or is trumped by another unexpected change. This could be seen as a failure of the treatment but equally, and possibly more fairly, as a temporary perturbation that should settle and allow nidotherapy to proceed later.

When no progress is being made on a nidopathway, when a planned change is recognised to be a wrong one, or when in other ways the ability to change things seems to have come to a standstill, it is reasonable to suspend nidotherapy, rather than abandoning it, as it can be resurrected at any time in the future.

How do you avoid bias in nidotherapy because the patient is listened to more than the other health professionals involved?

There is clearly a potential for bias that needs to be recognised in nidotherapy. However, most patients in a psychiatric service also feel there is a persistent bias against them and their voices are not easily heard. In this context the nidotherapist is a valuable ally and can redress the balance to some extent in their advocacy role. What must also be recognised is that an uncritical acceptance of the patients' opinions and wishes without taking into account

85

the views of other professionals is counterproductive, so regular feedback to clinical teams is an important, if sometimes under-emphasised, part of nidotherapy (see also Spencer *et al*, 2009).

How do you avoid exploitation of the nidotherapist by the patient?

Any therapist working singly with a patient can be exploited by, and/or exploit, the patient. It is not a reason for avoiding nidotherapy but it is a reminder that supervision and liaison are necessary before nidotherapy is set up.

When is the best time to end nidotherapy?

Because of pressures in all services, both public and private, there is a tendency to set the period of nidotherapy in advance. If time is important the full nidotherapy process can be completed in four sessions as described in chapter 9, but this would have to be associated with additional homework and exercises outside the therapy sessions. Ending can clearly be planned or unplanned, but as the intention is to make it a collaborative exercise it is much better to prepare the ground in advance.

Why does nidotherapy have to be separate from clinical teams? Why can't it be incorporated into the team structure?

We agree this is a difficult question. The best answer is a pragmatic one. There was no special attempt to keep nidotherapy distinct from the team when it was first tried but because it led to a certain amount of dissent and argument it was felt preferable to detach the service. The clear advantages of the nidotherapist acting as a confidante and advocate for the patient have been noted and these are seen as greater than those of integrating the therapist with the team. This does not mean that the nidotherapist always has to be kept separate from the main team providing therapy but this is probably the best starting point in treatment.

Do people have to understand nidotherapy in order to receive the treatment?

No. Although nidotherapy is a collaborative venture best carried out with the full involvement of the patient, it can be practised indirectly and by proxy. This applies particularly in people with severe intellectual disability, in whom the source of problem behaviours and symptoms may often have to be inferred.

Appendix
Answers to exercises

Exercise 2.1 (p. 23)

Question 1. Is this patient suitable for referral for nidotherapy?

The answer to this question is probably 'yes'. Some might argue that the diagnosis of paranoid schizophrenia is a strong possibility and that a full course of antipsychotic drug treatment possibly with additional psychological therapy such as cognitive–behavioural therapy is necessary before direct treatment options are abandoned. However, there is little to suggest that the patient might respond to this therapy and there is little chance that this would be adhered to even if it was given at first in adequate dosage under compulsion. The reasons for preferring nidotherapy at this stage are: (a) there is a clear environmental focus to the problem; (b) the obvious standard means of dealing with the problem have failed; and (c) if the environment was changed to the patient's satisfaction the clinical problem would, at least at this early stage in assessment, apparently be solved.

Question 2. What information is needed before nidotherapy can be started?

Close examination of the past history of the patient to determine whether any improvement has been shown with treatment in the past. This would give some clue as to whether direct treatment would be of benefit if given more energetically or from a different standpoint with regard to the patient's cooperation.

Question 3. What would be the essential elements that would need to be considered before taking him on for care?

Trust and openness. It is imperative that the potential nidotherapist is not seen as another health worker trying to 'diagnose the condition' but as someone who will, as dispassionately as possible, find out what changes are wanted by the patient and for all of these to be seriously considered. This can be gleaned to some extent from discussions with the clinicians who have already been involved in care, but really needs a preliminary face-to-face meeting at a place of the patient's choosing, very likely his home, to have an open discussion.

Exercise 3.1 (p. 30)

Question 1. How would you go about analysing Dwain's environmental needs in the light of his indifference to the environment?

This is not an easy task and there is more than one strategy that can be used. It is possible that Dwain will divulge more of what he really wants if the nidotherapist can get a little closer to understanding how he functions, what are his hopes and fears, and why he appears to have given up on any plans he had earlier in life. Exploration of his childhood and adolescence may be helpful here, mainly to find out about his interests at that time, who he may have admired or imitated, what goals he was aiming for in life, and what he did to try and achieve them. Interviews with members of his family and friends, preferably those with longer acquaintance, may also fill in the gaps for the nidotherapist.

Question 2. What degree of cooperation would you need from Dwain before you attempted to carry out a nidotherapy plan?

Nidotherapy is a cooperative exercise but Dwain probably comes into the group that is incapable of understanding the purpose of the intervention. He does not really recognise the problems he creates except at a very primitive level, and although this may change over the longer term, it is better for the nidotherapist to derive a plan from all the information available, asking Dwain to approve it in principle and making minor changes in conjunction with this. Collaboration does not end here; in subsequent sessions Dwain can be asked for his own feedback on progress and this can influence the course of change. It would be a mistake to finish the attempt to effect any form of change because Dwain is not able to cooperate or reflect on what might be needed.

Exercise 4.1 (p. 36)

The supervisor and nidotherapist need to follow the advice given in Box 4.2 (p. 34) before deciding how to proceed. The nidotherapist is usually in the best position to decide whether the request by the patient to be accompanied to the job centre is an appropriate one or not. It is reasonable to expect that the interview will be an anxiety-provoking occasion and the presence of the nidotherapist could be of great value, but the request could also indicate a degree of dependence or attachment that could be counterproductive. The supervisor, either from direct discussion or with feedback from others, may be able to advise whether the relationship between patient and therapist is either going beyond or could be construed as going beyond acceptable boundaries, and this deserves to be discussed openly. A balance has to be struck between the clear wish of both patient and therapist to make the best use of a potentially more favourable environment, and the possible handicaps. The risks are best examined by close study of past behaviour – if all the episodes of past sex offending have taken place when the patient has been under the influence of alcohol this may be reassuring, but it also

Exercise 4.1 *(contd)*

may be true that the wishes are present on many more occasions and are only transferred into action after the disinhibition created by the effects of alcohol. In the last resort the nidotherapist has to ask herself 'Is this a reasonable request and would I accede to it if it was put to me by somebody else in a similar position?' If it is considered reasonable, and the patient has a clear indication of the specific role of the therapist at the job centre, then the decision would be to agree with the request, as to do otherwise could be construed as discrimination. However, if the reason for the request was construed as merely an attempt to establish a closer relationship and the presence of the therapist as a professional adviser was not deemed to be the real purpose of the request, it could be rejected.

Exercise 5.1 (p. 41)

Question 1. Formulate a nidopathway, including its planned length, which would enable Margery to live away from her family.

A full assessment should be made of Margery's wishes and abilities to live independently and the level of support she needs. If there was a mismatch between her abilities and her wishes, the possibility of shared accommodation or a related arrangement should be considered. Once the requirements have been agreed by both nidotherapist and patient the plan needs to be approved by the eating disorders team and modified if necessary but only with the patient's approval. The timescale for both the placement and the transfer date need to be planned with the eating disorders team.

Question 2. What should her family be told about this plan, and should it be the responsibility of the clinical team or the nidotherapist?

The clinical team in the eating disorders service should inform the family members about the assessment and its purpose. Their anxieties may be allayed by a regular bulletin on progress. It would be unwise for the nidotherapist to be in contact with the family unless and until the patient feels confident enough for contact to be established.

Question 3. How frequently would the nidopathway be monitored and what should be the plan if there seems to be evidence of the symptoms and behaviour of her eating disorder returning?

The frequency of monitoring by the eating disorders team is determined primarily by them but the nidotherapist should have some say in this in an advocacy role for the patient. The criteria for relapse would be those normally adopted by the clinical team and would also be known by the nidotherapist and patient. There could be some latitude in their interpretation in which the nidotherapist could play a part too.

Exercise 9.1 (p. 70)

The answer follows the five sections from the first stage of nidotherapy discussed in chapter 9. What is clear at the beginning is that treatment will take much longer than a single session to complete.

1. Developing a trusting relationship with the patient as a person in his own preferred setting

Two questions are in the background in this part of the assessment, and indeed will have been asked many times previously in this phase: 'Would this person remain well if he avoided cannabis altogether, with or without some antipsychotic medication for schizophrenic symptoms?', 'Is their any prospect of either of these being accepted voluntarily by the patient?' The answers are not going to be gained from a formal interview, for example in a psychiatric ward, and doubtless they have been asked in this setting on many occasions previously. The nidotherapist needs to stress his or her independence from the others who have been involved previously, and to see the patient in the most positive environment possible for disclosure, most likely at home. This will not be an easy set of interviews, and the nidotherapist will have to be as receptive and non-judgemental as possible to get answers that will help him or her make the decision.

2. Determining which of the current problems are linked to the environment

The most obvious targets here are the environmental factors that might lie behind the taking of cannabis and, because of the history of the problem, whether there are sets of circumstances in which social anxiety is less or absent. Social anxiety appears to be a likely precursor of cannabis consumption but careful elucidation of its exact relationship to the cannabis will be needed. Finding situations in which the man is in tune with his life to the extent that cannabis is not needed may also help in planning nidotherapy.

3. Analysis of environmental needs

There is an important distinction between demands (or wants) and needs. In the words of Stevens and Gabbay (1991) '"need" may best be defined as the ability to benefit from "healthcare", which depends both on morbidity and on the effectiveness of care. An analysis of its relationship with "demand", which is the healthcare that people ask for, and "supply", which is provided, exposes the limitations of current information sources, and confirms that the formal assessment of needs will inevitably be a lengthy task'. In this man's current thinking processes the provision of cannabis is a need, but officially it fails, as do all addictions, because it leads to no benefit to health. It is a major task to convert this demand into a recognisable need that does confer benefit. Nidotherapy has the potential to do this by shifting the focus from the drug to the environment that creates the demand.

4. Assessment of changes necessary to achieve environmental needs

At this stage it is too much to expect to get more than a rough idea of the changes that may be necessary. What is required is the recognition that changes are feasible provided the other elements are in position.

Exercise 9.1 *(contd)*

5. Integration of needs

By the end of this stage it is helpful to have one or two (at the most) coherent themes to bring forward to the later stages. The alternative is a set of unconnected environmental suggestions that may be difficult to implement in a common plan.

Exercise 9.2 (pp. 71–72)

Again it is useful to follow the checklist in planning this exercise.

1. Provisional pathway

At every session build in time to find out what has happened since the last visit. This may not appear too difficult on the surface, but it is important not to take everything at face value. It is possible that a move to better accommodation is just a smokescreen hiding another problem or environmental deficiency which needs exposing. Does she make any effort to move? Has she planned for a move or is she dreading it? Find out and explore.

2. Environmental testing and planned environmental change

This is difficult to anticipate, but there may be many opportunities for a change in housing to be tested for a short time only before making a final decision to continue this path.

The solution to the main problems may appear to be a clear one: to do everything possible to effect a housing move to a better location. In moving forward with this it is important for the nidotherapist to take a broader view of the problem and not just act as a highly energetic and effective housing support worker. The depression and other psychiatric symptoms are unlikely to disappear overnight if the right accommodation is found, and as every move to new accommodation is a stressful and sometimes lonely experience, the depression and paranoia could be aggravated even after a move to apparently ideal accommodation. There are also family members who are of great potential help but who are likely to be wary of becoming involved. The nidotherapist could be an essential go-between who can reconcile differences and allow more support to be given in both planning and effecting the preferred changes.

3. Person feedback

Good nidotherapists are expected to be sensible, organised people who act efficiently and effectively as personal, social and physical environmental problem solvers. By the end of this phase they could be forgiven for pressing on with a plan that has the tacit approval of the patient, who by now is taking a back seat in the negotiations – but they shouldn't be allowed to do this! Before deciding on the

Exercise 9.2 *(contd)*

plan everything needs to have been discussed fully with the patient and all possible obstacles and tripwires explored. Join with the patient's uncertainty about the way to go – say how anxious you would feel and how you would cope with this. A set of questions beginning 'What would you do if…?' should be put before the patient before any plan is decided and, where necessary, the strategies derived from this incorporated into the plan.

4. Formulation of the final pathway

The final planned pathway can be a general verbal agreement or a carefully written document, but the essentials must be clear before it is implemented in any way. Not every problem can be anticipated but it is important that the core components are agreed, and for these to remain in place even if there are hiccoughs along the way. It may also be helpful to have a stopping point decided before the plan is implemented. If a set of requirements is not achieved or if the environmental factors change dramatically, when should the plan be abandoned or changed? Both nidotherapist and patient should be agreed on when these points are reached but this should be a general agreement only; if the right degree of trust is present the details will look after themselves.

Exercise 9.3 (p. 76)

Question: Describe how you would monitor the nidopathway and Malcolm's depression in a way that could satisfy the hypothesis that his work style was the main factor reinforcing his depression.

The straightforward scientific method would be to rate Malcolm's depression and the progress with his llama farming and to hope for a strong negative correlation between his depression levels and llama success. However, this almost certainly will not be necessary and may be confusing. The right way forward is to warn Malcolm that at the beginning of this exercise there will be anxieties and doubts and it is unlikely that his depression will suddenly change to persistent optimism. But if he has got it right, his mood will lift as the challenge gets under way and he sees the other advantages of having llamas (e.g. they keep the foxes at bay). The link between his mood and farming success is likely to be a stuttering one and may fail, but this will be a very valuable environmental experiment that should help to find further ways forward.

References

Abrahamson, S. (2007) Did Janet Frame have high-functioning autism? *New Zealand Medical Journal*, **120**, U2747.

Alexander, F. (1930) The neurotic character. *International Journal of Psychoanalysis*, **11**, 291–311.

Barrett, R. J. (1996) *The Psychiatric Team and the Social Definition of Schizophrenia: An Anthropological Study of Person and Illness*. Cambridge University Press.

Bateman, A. & Zanarini, M. (2008) Personality disorders. In: *The Cambridge Textbook of Effective Treatment in Psychiary* (ed P. Tyrer & K. R. Silk), pp. 659–681. Cambridge University Press.

Berrios, G. (2008) The history of psychiatric therapies. In: *The Cambridge Textbook of Effective Treatment in Psychiary* (ed P. Tyrer & K. R. Silk), pp. 16–43. Cambridge University Press.

Brown, G. & Harris, T. (1978) *The Social Origins of Depression*. Tavistock Publications.

Brown, J., Simons, L. & Zeeman, L. (2008) New ways of working: how mental health practitioners perceive their training and role. *Journal of Psychiatric Mental Health Nursing*, **15**, 823–832.

Burns, T., Creed, F., Fahy, T., *et al* (1999) Intensive versus standard case management for severe psychotic illness: a randomised trial. *Lancet*, **353**, 2185–2189.

Cawley, R. H. (1993) Psychiatry is more than a science. *British Journal of Psychiatry*, **162**, 154–160.

Clark, C. L. (2000) *Social Work Ethics: Politics, Principles and Practice*. Palgrave Macmillan.

Cohen, P. (2006) *Change in Personality Status in a Long Term Cohort of Children in the Community*. Paper presented at 7th European Congress of the International Society for the Study of Personality Disorders, Prague, June 2006.

Costa, P. T. & McCrae, R. R. (1992) *The NEO–PI–R: Professional Manual. Revised NEO Personality Inventory (NEO–PI–R) and NEO Five Factor Inventory (NEO–FFI)*. Psychological Assessment Resources.

Craddock, N. & Owen, M. J. (2005) The beginning of the end for the Kraepelinian dichotomy. *British Journal of Psychiatry*, **186**, 364–366.

Crawford, T. N., Cohen, P., First, M. B., *et al* (2008a) Comorbid Axis I and Axis II disorders in early adolescence: outcomes 20 years later. *Archives of General Psychiatry*, **65**, 641–648.

Crawford, M. J., Price, K., Rutter, D., *et al* (2008b) Dedicated community-based services for adults with personality disorder: Delphi study. *British Journal of Psychiatry*, **193**, 342–343.

Darwin, C. (1859) *The Origin of Species*. Reprinted 1970 (Everyman edn), Dent.

Dawkins, R. (2006) *The Selfish Gene (3rd edn)*. Oxford University Press.

Eliot., T. S. (1917) *The Love Song of J. Alfred Prufrock*. Amereon.

Evans, S., Huxley, P., Gately, C., *et al* (2006) Mental health, burnout and job satisfaction among mental health social workers in England and Wales. *British Journal of Psychiatry*, **188**, 75–80.

Frame, J. (2001) *An Angel at My Table: The Complete Autobiography*. The Women's Press.

Garety, P. A., Fowler, D. G., Freeman, D., *et al* (2008) Cognitive–behavioural therapy and family intervention for relapse prevention and symptom reduction in psychosis: randomised controlled trial. *British Journal of Psychiatry*, **192**, 412–423.

Hare, R. D. (1991) *The Hare Psychopathy Checklist – Revised*. Multi-Health Systems.

Harrison-Read, P., Lucas, B., Tyrer, P., *et al* (2002) Heavy users of acute psychiatric beds: randomised controlled trial of enhanced community management in an outer London borough. *Psychological Medicine*, **32**, 413–426.

Holloway, F. (2008) Is there a science of recovery and does it matter? *Advances in Psychiatric Treatment*, **14**, 245–247.

Huxley, A. (1932) *Brave New World*. Reprinted 2004. Vintage.

Killaspy, H., Bebbington, P., Blizard, R., *et al* (2006) The REACT study: randomised evaluation of assertive community treatment in north London. *BMJ*, **332**, 815–820.

Kingdon, D. G. & Turkington, D. (1995) *Cognitive–Behavioural Therapy of Schizophrenia*. Brunner-Routledge.

Leff, J., Kuipers, L. & Berkowitz, R. (1982) A controlled trial of social intervention in the families of schizophrenic patients. *British Journal of Psychiatry*, **141**, 121–134.

Leff, J., Kuipers, L., Berkowitz, R., *et al* (1985) A controlled trial of social intervention in the families of schizophrenic patients: two year follow-up. *British Journal of Psychiatry*, **146**, 594–600.

Leucht, S., Corves, C., Arbter, D., *et al* (2009) Second-generation versus first-generation antipsychotic drugs for schizophrenia: a meta-analysis. *Lancet*, **373**, 31–41.

Marriott, S., Malone, S., Onyett, S., *et al* (1993) The consequences of an open referral system to a community mental health service. *Acta Psychiatrica Scandinavica*, **88**, 93–97.

Marx, A. J., Test, M. A. & Stein, L. I. (1973) Extra-hospital management of severe mental illness: feasibility and effects of social functioning. *Archives of General Psychiatry*, **29**, 505–511.

Meagher, D. J., O'Hanlon, D., O'Mahony, E., *et al* (1996) The use of environmental strategies and psychotropic medication in the management of delirium. *British Journal of Psychiatry*, **168**, 512–515.

Mountain, D. & Shah, P. J. (2008) Recovery and the medical model. *Advances in Psychiatric Treatment*, **14**, 241–244.

Newton-Howes, G., Tyrer, P. & Johnson, T. (2006) Personality disorder and the outcome of depression: meta-analysis of published studies. *British Journal of Psychiatry*, **188**, 13–20.

Owen, D. (2008) *The Hubris Syndrome: Bush, Blair and the Intoxication of Power*. Politico's Publishing.

Pollitt, J. D. (1960) Depression and the functional shift. *Comprehensive Psychiatry*, **1**, 381–90.

Ranger, M., Methuen, C., Rutter D, *et al* (2004) Prevalence of personality disorder in the caseload of an inner city assertive outreach team. *Psychiatric Bulletin*, **28**, 441–443.

Ranger, M., Tyrer, P., Miloseska, K., *et al* (2009) Cost-effectiveness of nidotherapy for comorbid personality disorder and severe mental illness: randomized controlled trial. *Epidemiologia e Psichiatria Sociale*, **18**, 128–136.

Resnick, S. G., Rosenheck, R. A. & Lehman, A. F. (2004) An exploratory analysis of correlates of recovery. *Psychiatric Services*, **55**, 540–547.

Sargant, W. (1966) Psychiatric treatment in general teaching hospitals: a plea for a mechanistic approach. *BMJ*, **2**, 257–262.

Scott, J. (2008) Cognitive–behavioural therapy for severe mental disorders: back to the future? *British Journal of Psychiatry*, **192**, 401–403.

Shine, J. & Hobson, J. (2000) Institutional behaviour and time in treatment among psychopaths admitted to a prison-based therapeutic community. *Medicine, Science and Law*, **40**, 327–335.

Spencer, S.-J., Rutter, D. & Tyrer, P. (2009) Integration of nidotherapy into the management of mental illness and antisocial personality: a qualitative study. *International Journal of Social Psychiatry*, **55** (in press).

Stein, L. I. & Santos, A. B. (1998) *Assertive Community Treatment of Persons with Severe Mental Illness*. WW Norton.

Stevens, A. & Gabbay, J. (1991) Needs assessment needs assessment. *Health Trends*, **23**, 20–23.

Tarrier, N., Wittkowski, A., Kinney, C., *et al* (1999) Durability of the effects of cognitive–behavioural therapy in the treatment of chronic schizophrenia: 12-month follow-up. *British Journal of Psychiatry*, **174**, 500–504.

Thornicroft, G. & Tansella, M. (2004) Components of a modern mental health service: a pragmatic balance of community and hospital care: overview of systematic evidence. *British Journal of Psychiatry*, **185**, 283–290.

Tyrer, P. (2002) Nidotherapy: a new approach to the treatment of personality disorder. *Acta Psychiatrica Scandinavica*, **105**, 469–471.

Tyrer, P. (2003) *How to Cope with Stress (2nd edn)*. Sheldon Press.

Tyrer, P. (2007) Personality diatheses: a superior description than disorder. *Psychological Medicine*, **37**, 1521–1525.

Tyrer, P. (2008) Personality disorder and public mental health. *Clinical Medicine*, **8**, 423–427.

Tyrer, P. & Bajaj, P. (2005) Nidotherapy: making the environment do the therapeutic work. *Advances in Psychiatric Treatment*, **11**, 232–238.

Tyrer, P. & Kramo, K. (2007) Nidotherapy in practice. *Journal of Mental Health*, **16**, 117–131.

Tyrer, P. & Steinberg, D. (2005) The Social Model. In *Models for Mental Disorder* (4th edn), pp. 99–114. Wiley.

Tyrer, P., Kramo, K., Miloseska, K., *et al* (2007) The place for nidotherapy in psychiatric practice. *Psychiatric Bulletin*, **31**, 1–3.

Wessely, S., Hotopf, M. & Sharpe, M. (1998) *Chronic Fatigue and its Syndromes*, pp. 324–332. Oxford University Press.

Willi, J. (1999) *Ecological Psychotherapy: Developing by Shaping the Personal Niche*. Seattle, Hogrefe & Huber.

Index

Compiled by Caroline Sheard